Skills Training for Struggling Kids

Skills Training
for Struggling Kids

Promoting Your Child's
Behavioral, Emotional, Academic,
and Social Development

Michael L. Bloomquist, PhD

THE GUILFORD PRESS
New York   London

Library of Congress Cataloging-in-Publication Data

Bloomquist, Michael L.
    Skills training for struggling kids : promoting your child's behavioral, emotional, academic, and social development / by Michael L. Bloomquist.
        p.   cm.
    Includes bibliographical references and index.
    ISBN 978-1-60918-170-3 (pbk. : alk. paper)
    1. Problem children—Behavior modification.   2. Problem children—
Education.   3. Behavior disorders in children—Treatment.   4. Parenting.   I. Title.
    HQ773.B56 2013
    618.92'89—dc23
                                                                2012028854

To my wife, Rebecca

Contents

Acknowledgments

Many people helped me in writing the "Struggling Kids" books, and I am most indebted to them. I am forever grateful for the love and support of my wife, Rebecca Syverts, who is always there for me. I thank Steve Schnell and Marcia Jensen for early helpful ideas and comments that shaped the focus of the books. I am very appreciative of the feedback and guidance of Kitty Moore, Executive Editor, and Christine Benton, Developmental Editor, both at The Guilford Press. Lastly, to the many families with whom I have had the privilege to work over the years and who have taught me so much, I want to express my sincere gratitude.

Skills Training for Struggling Kids

Introduction
How to Use This Book

This book is for parents seeking practical and effective strategies to help a child[1] who is experiencing behavioral-emotional problems. This book is for you if your child is struggling to function adequately at home, at school, or with friends. It's for you if your child is struggling with negative or overwhelming feelings or lack of confidence. If you have a struggling child, you are undoubtedly worried, and your inability to get your child back on track on your own may also have left you exasperated and exhausted. You need tried-and-true solutions to help the child you care about so much.

In the following pages you'll find a wide variety of solutions for a diverse range of behavioral–emotional problems experienced by children ages 5–17. The strategies and insights offered here, derived from nearly 25 years of my work with children and families in both practice and research settings, will help your child build the skills necessary to master the tasks of childhood and proceed along a productive developmental path. Although the ideas and procedures described will not necessarily make everything better, there is still reason for optimism: The research shows that building these skills produces effective results when the strategies are well implemented, and I have personally seen countless families make enormous progress.

Faithfully following the instructions and sticking with the program are, however, essential. For this reason, **you will get the most out of this book if you work with a trained practitioner who has experience with these methods and is using the accompanying practitioner manual.** A qualified practitioner can help you devise a plan for helping your child build skills that will, in turn, help him or her overcome any particular struggles. In addition, the practitioner can then coach you in learning the strategies laid out in this book. You will then be applying these strategies at home, so the explanations, instructions, and tips you find in the following

---

[1]The term *child* is used generically throughout the book and generally applies to children and teens.

chapters have been written so that you can easily refer back to the instructions and use them when a practitioner is not right there with you. Many parents find, in fact, that the methods are so straightforward that they can learn to use them without a practitioner. If you glance through this book and feel that you can tackle the work on your own, then the greatest strength of this book for you may be that you have so many options of skills-building strategies to try. You can always seek professional help down the road if you hit a snag. The companion practitioner volume that parallels this book can be used by a professional you consult to ensure that you're all working with the same methods, toward the same goals.

The Struggling Child

Here are the stories of two children and their parents. These composites of real people represent children and their families who are trying their best every day. You may identify with some of their trials and tribulations.

William's Story

William is 10 years old and sometimes "forgets" to do what he's told. With reminders, however, he typically follows directions, whether he's at home with his mom, Shauna, at his dad Rick's apartment, or in his fifth-grade classroom. He was lucky to have his learning problems spotted during first grade, so he's pretty much kept pace with the other kids his age, thanks to special education classes in reading and math. At first the other kids made fun of him for having to leave his classroom and go to the "dummy's" reading group, but William's parents told him to shrug off the teasing, and they gave him some good one-liners to toss back at his classmates.

Even though William has had troubles, he's also experienced his share of triumphs. This year he was elected student council representative for his classroom. When there's a problem to be solved, many kids go to William, because he always tells them to "chill out" and try to work out any problems they are having.

William isn't going to win any awards for his athletic ability, but his Little League coach says he's the anchor of the team—the player who supports everyone else and always cheers the loudest. The day he struck out and "lost the game for the team," he felt so humiliated that he phoned his dad—and then ended up talking himself out of skipping the next practice!

William loves to sing in the church choir, where he sometimes has trouble sticking to the program and has been labeled the "class clown" of the group. He knows to excuse himself for a few minutes when he feels like he just can't stand still a second longer, so now he's not breaking up the rehearsals as he did before.

At the year's first parent–teacher conference William's fifth-grade teacher describes him as "a joy to have in class" and says "he has good ideas." Shauna and Rick express concern that he's still only a C student. They agree to keep in close touch with the teacher. They plan to give William some extra homework assignments that might boost his proficiency in specific math concepts and also to take out library books recommended for boys his age. Since Shauna and Rick are divorced, they plan on coordinating this effort across their respective homes.

Jessica's Story

Jessica doesn't follow instructions, and her parents are frustrated. It's very tiring to have to tell her over and over what to do, whether it's to get ready for bed, finish her homework, clean up after herself, or even turn off the TV. Just about everything is an argument with Jessica, and it shouldn't have to be this way. She is, after all, 14.

The problem isn't limited to home either, and now Samantha and Bob are being forced to deal with phone calls from their daughter's teachers, who have numerous complaints: Jessica can't seem to pay attention without constant reminders; she disrupts the class by talking incessantly; she stares out the window or doodles instead of completing class work. Jessica's grades, the teachers warn, are taking a nosedive.

Jessica's struggles are not new. She has always been what the books label "the difficult child." Even as a baby she was fussy and irritable, and her toddler and preschool years were marked by difficulty getting along with peers. Ever since early grade school, Jessica's teachers have reported that she is frequently off task and disruptive in the classroom. However, Jessica has experienced times during which she has done okay. But Samantha and Bob notice that, overall, Jessica's problems are gradually getting worse rather than better.

Recently Samantha and Bob tried talking to Jessica to see if they could help her, but Jessica only sits there looking sullen. When they pause to ask if she's listening, she snaps at them or bursts into tears and runs out. Samantha and Bob have even tried to elicit help from her much-adored older brother, Danny, but she won't even let Danny into her room or her life. Jessica has clammed up. She gives only one-word replies to her parents' or brother's tentative questions at the dinner table and seems to avoid her family whenever possible. The once chatty girl rarely volunteers her thoughts or feelings or shares stories about what's going on in her life. She seems sad and preoccupied much of the time.

Jessica's parents comfort themselves with the idea that it's typical teenage angst and the hope that she's switched her alliance from family to friends. It's only normal, they tell each other. But they know it's not. When the phone rings in the evening, it's always for Danny. When they catch a glimpse of the kids waiting for the school bus in the morning, Jessica is always off by herself. All the tests show that Jessica has above-average intelligence, but because of the drop in her academic performance, they are evaluating her to see if she might qualify for an individualized education program (IEP) at school.

Samantha and Bob know that their daughter has a lot to offer the world. She draws beautifully and is a decent soccer player. But as of late her sketchpads have been gathering dust in the corner of her room, and she's no longer a starter in soccer because she's "hard to coach." She's struggling in every aspect of her life, and her parents are heartbroken. They're desperate to find a way to get Jessica back on track.

In many ways William and Jessica are typical of children who experience problems as they grow up. William's difficulties appear to be less serious than Jessica's, perhaps because he exhibits the skills to overcome some of his problems and shows that he has already mastered a lot of developmental tasks in spite of his learning problems. He has learned some skills of emotional control and of social problem solving, and his family members show a strong ability to work together to help him keep building skills in all domains of his life. This book focuses on the children who have behavioral and emotional problems that are similar to William's and Jessica's and shows you how to help your own child develop skills to overcome these problems, just like William.

The Characteristics of a Struggling Child

William and Jessica are both examples of a struggling child. In this book the term *struggling child* is used to describe a youngster who is exhibiting behaviors and emotional responses that are disruptive, aggressive, volatile, moody, or worrisome, to name a few possibilities. Unfortunately, these behavioral–emotional problems negatively affect a child's everyday functioning, which in turn typically stresses out parents and other family members. The struggling child is often "behind" in behavioral, social, emotional, and academic areas of psychological development. The well-being of parents and families with a struggling child is sometimes less than optimal too. If left unchecked, the problems of a struggling child can worsen over time and have harmful long-term effects on the family as well. The characteristics of the struggling child are detailed in Chapter 1.

How to Help a Struggling Child

The problems of struggling children can seem overwhelming at times, as they were beginning to feel for Jessica's parents. Nonetheless, there is a lot that can be done to turn a struggling child around. A developmental skills enhancement approach, such as the one provided in this book, can be used to assist children in "catching up" to their peers in a psychological and developmental sense. This progress then leads to more success at home and school and with peers and to feeling better about themselves. In addition, family members can learn skills to help them cope better, thus leading to enhanced parent and family functioning.

One way to think about how this turnaround is accomplished is to think in terms of how children learn skills naturally, as they develop, and how this learning impacts parents and the rest of the family. Most children learn behavioral, social, emotional, and academic skills through everyday life experiences. For whatever reason, struggling children have not learned these important skills satisfactorily, which hampers their ability to succeed at home, at school, and with friends. Much like a child with a speech articulation problem, who has to be taught how to pronounce words that others have learned naturally, the struggling child has to be explicitly taught behavioral, social, emotional, and academic skills. And the child's skills-building and developmental progress will always be enhanced by having parents who can manage stress, cope with adult personal and family life, and model all the behavioral and emotional skills their children need to learn. A struggling child who receives explicit skills-building instruction and receives all the support and aid that devoted parents can give, will likely discover a new road to everyday success. William and Jessica, and their families, would benefit from learning developmental and coping skills to get back on track. The basics of the skills-building approach are presented in Chapters 1 and 2 and elaborated throughout this book.

The "Struggling Kids" Skills-Building Program

Skills Training for Struggling Kids and the companion *Practitioner Guide* are based in part on a revision of the book, *Skills Training for Children with Behavior Problems,* published in 2006. The new volumes have been updated and reorganized to add skills-training procedures, to place a greater emphasis on making sure that parents and children get off to a good start and follow through, and to facilitate practitioners' work with families. It's my hope that these enhancements will make the material even more useful to both parents and practitioners with a wide range of needs.

The parent and practitioner books comprise a coordinated curriculum that is hereafter referred to simply as the "Struggling Kids" program. This program is designed to aid parents and practitioners in their efforts to work together collaboratively to get a struggling child and a stressed-out family back on track. You can use this book on your own if you feel confident in following the instructions and sticking to the methods. Or, as part of the overall program designed for use by practitioners, this book can be used in individual or group training sessions with the professional, and as a reference for home use when building and practicing the new skills.

The Focus of the "Struggling Kids" Program

Although the program is aimed mostly at the child or teen (ages 5–17 years), you, the parent, are the primary recipient of this skills-building approach because you have the most influence over your child's development. **In this program you will learn new skills and learn how to guide your child and family to use them.** Many of the ideas and procedures described in the "Struggling Kids" program involve either parents changing their behavior or parents assisting their child to make behavior changes. Research, experience, and knowledge of child development confirm that helping you help your struggling child is almost always the best approach.

The Methods Used in the "Struggling Kids" Program

The ideas and procedures in the "Struggling Kids" program are based on research showing that skills-building interventions work. They are derived from behavioral therapy techniques that have been tested thoroughly and proven effective when implemented well. That is, the research showing this approach is effective when involved families work with well-trained and qualified practitioners. For this reason, and because trained professionals can guide you through the twists and turns you're likely to encounter in trying to implement the strategies with your own family, you are likely to see maximum improvement if you work with a practitioner who has expertise and experience in child and family behavioral therapy.

An Overview of the Parent Book

The book is broadly written for a *parent*, meaning any adult in a caregiver role with a child, and a *family*, which includes any primary living arrangement(s) for a child.

The term *child* is used generically throughout to indicate children ages 5–17 years. There are suggestions for adjusting the strategies for a younger child, an older child, or a teen. All ideas and skills presented are equally applicable to males and females. Since every family is unique, a one-size-fits-all approach is not used. **Rather, you are encouraged to tailor your efforts—with the guidance of this book alone or in collaboration with a practitioner—and select skills-building strategies that fit your child's age, the unique circumstances of your family, and the goals you are trying to achieve.**

What You Will Find in the Pages Ahead

This book provides information and skills-building strategies to promote your child's success and your family's ability to cope. In a nutshell the topics covered include:

- Up-to-date information on behavioral–emotional problems in children.

- Conceiving of a child's struggles as setbacks in development.

- Viewing parenting and family problems as setbacks in coping with stress.

- Getting motivated and following through to make meaningful changes.

- Skills-building strategies to develop a child's behavioral, social, emotional, and academic skills.

- Skills-building strategies to improve a parent's coping and broader family interactions.

Each of these topics is summarized briefly in Chapters 1–3 and then elaborated throughout the book. Chapters 4–20 provide step-by-step instructions for using effective skills-building strategies. You can learn the strategies by reading the instructions, doing some role plays to "rehearse" the methods and see how they might work for your family, and then start applying them on a regular basis to build the skills. Alternatively, a practitioner can help you learn the strategies, advise you on how to practice them at home, and help you surmount any obstacles you encounter. The skills-building chapters also illustrate typical behavioral–emotional struggles and the use of particular strategies and troubleshooting approaches that will prove helpful when you're not making the progress you'd like to make. Each of these chapters will give you the knowledge and practical strategies to solve problems and promote optimal development in your child and enhance family relationships. This "Struggling Kids" program uses a positive and optimistic approach that is based on the assumptions that your child can learn concrete skills to boost competence and that you can learn skills to improve your own and your family's well-being.

A Toolbox Approach

Although I refer to "Struggling Kids" as a program and a curriculum, it might be best to view this book as a *toolbox* containing numerous tools that you can use to get your child and family back on course. There are checklists, charts, and worksheets in each chapter to aid in learning, practicing, and monitoring the progress of your skills-building efforts. Some charts are visually oriented to illustrate skills for children of all ages. Readers have permission, and are encouraged, to make copies of the charts to use.

How to Use This Parent Book

When someone hands you a toolbox, how do you know which tool to use and when? This book is not intended to be read from cover to cover. In fact, it would be unnecessary and impossible to do everything described. Obviously, therefore, you need to figure out which skills you and your child need to build and in what order. If, after reading the first three chapters, you have any doubts about what to tackle and in what order, a competent practitioner who has experience in child and family behavioral therapy can be very valuable. In that case, you and your family's practitioner can collaborate in devising a plan for using the book and then carrying out the skills-building methods.

I also encourage you to read this book in an exploratory fashion to get an idea of what options are available to you. Read through the information-focused Chapters 1–3 to find out the best way to develop a plan of action, set goals, and get motivated. You can then select one or several skills-focused chapters at first and others later on.

Because all of the skills-building strategies are geared to different target areas that emerge over time, **this book can be used throughout the course of your child's development, and it can be used with different children in your family if the need arises.**

Please be aware that, even when you work hard at using the skills-building strategies in this book, your child may need additional support and help. Some children have behavioral–emotional problems that are serious enough to warrant additional mental health, educational, juvenile justice, and/or other community services. Indeed research shows that combinations of different interventions typically work better than one intervention alone. A qualified practitioner can coordinate any other services that may be needed.

Skills Training for Struggling Kids is not intended to substitute for evaluation and treatment services provided by qualified healthcare professionals.

The Author's Hope

It is my hope that this book and the skills-building strategies described in it will help your child and family reach important goals and succeed in many areas of life. I wish you and your family the very best!

Getting Started
and Staying with It

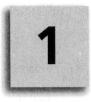

The Struggling Child

Understanding Your Child's Behavioral–Emotional Problems

Child difficulties like disrupting the classroom, arguing with adults, fighting with siblings, moodiness, excessive worrying, rejection by peers, and/or underachieving in school, to name just a few, are indicators of behavioral–emotional problems. Such behaviors and/or emotional symptoms can harm your child's functioning in everyday life, which in turn stresses you out and probably has a negative effect on family life. You are likely reading this book and perhaps working with a practitioner due to similar concerns and out of a desire to get your child and family back on track.

To do that you need to develop a specific plan of action that is exactly what your son or daughter needs to be successful (see Chapter 2). But first you have to understand your child's behavioral–emotional problems and begin thinking of them from a developmental point of view.

Understanding Your Child's Behavioral–Emotional Problems

Almost all children demonstrate the problems described in this section, to some extent. It is the **frequency** and **magnitude** of the problems that make the difference between a normal bump in the road and something to be concerned about. For example, habitual defiance is much more frequent than average and is a concern. A child who throws a chair while being defiant is demonstrating a problem behavior of much greater magnitude than run-of-the-mill talking back. Determining whether a child has crossed the line in frequency and magnitude for a particular problem is, unfortunately, a judgment call that is tough for many parents to make. This is where a qualified practitioner can help. Experienced practitioners have seen many children with problems and are also well versed in the symptoms of behavioral–emotional problems and when they should be addressed.

Following is a list of common characteristics of children that are problematic when their frequency and magnitude are high:

- **Hyperactivity**—can't sit still and is constantly in motion.

- **Impulsivity**—fails to think before acting, exhibits behavior such as blurting out, shoving in line, or even stealing something tempting.

- **Inattention**—is distracted, has difficulty focusing, and demonstrates low effort and motivation to complete tasks and stay focused.

- **Defiance**—argues with or disregards adult directives.

- **Rule-violating behavior**—violates commonly accepted standards of behavior such as breaking curfew, stealing, vandalizing, running away from home, skipping school.

- **Aggression**—displays actions that harm or intimidate another—*physical aggression*, like punching, hitting, and kicking, or *relational aggression*, like spreading rumors or excluding someone from a group—both of which can be expressed as *reactive* (spur of the moment) or *proactive* (planned).

- **Moodiness**—exhibits depression-like sadness, discouragement, and hopelessness; and/or euphoric excitability, mania, or irritability.

- **Anxiety**—worries, is physically tense, and avoids certain places, people, or events because of nervousness.

- **Emotionally overreactive**—acts aroused, agitated, and "ready for action."

- **Emotionally underreactive**—acts calm, with low guilt and/or concern for others (sometimes with lower empathy).

- **Underachievement**—experiences delays in reading, arithmetic, written language, and other areas of academic proficiency.

- **Social difficulties**—has a hard time with friends and peer interactions, possibly including being socially troublesome to others and/or withdrawn and shy.

These behavioral–emotional problems can all range from mild to severe, and some children may have more than one of them. It is unfortunately all too common that a child starts out with one or two of these problems, which lead to setbacks in everyday life, and then they "snowball," creating more problems over time. Although there are gender differences in the incidence of some of these problems, both boys and girls can exhibit any of them.

These behavioral–emotional problems may be the reasons you have sought assistance for your child, as they are for many parents. More often than not, these problems end up being the "target" of an intervention. It's essential, though, that you accurately identify the problems your child is experiencing before deciding what kind of help he or she needs. Here too a practitioner can help guide you.

Understanding Your Child's Developmental Struggles

The underlying premise of the "Struggling Kids" program is that a child with behavioral–emotional problems like the ones listed above is struggling with psychological development. That is, the child is behind in accumulating typical skills, or competencies, in the behavioral, social, emotional, and academic arenas. This is why the "Struggling Kids" program focuses on skills building: To be successful, the struggling child needs to be given the ability to master tasks that are part of typical child development.

To get a better idea of where your child stands in psychological development, review the ***Child Psychological Development*** chart. Compare the struggling and successful child in each area. Try to pinpoint your child's developmental progress. Is your child behind and struggling or on track and successful? Keep in mind that although your child may be at a certain chronological age (e.g., elementary school age), he or she may be at a younger developmental age (e.g., preschool), and if so, that means that your child is behind. If you're not sure where your child fits on the developmental path for any domain, try to think of examples of your child's behavior that prompt you to say that your child is struggling; a practitioner can guide you, if you need additional expertise in this area.

Child Psychological Development

Child Behavioral Development: Learning to follow reasonable external directions and rules and to internalize a moral and honest code of conduct

Age	Struggling child	Successful child
Infant/toddler	Irritable/fussy and/or unresponsive to parent.	Easygoing and responsive to parent.
	Often tantrums and whines.	Manageable "terrible 2's."

Age	Struggling child	Successful child
Preschool	Often disobeys caregiver's directions. Often violates house rules.	Usually obeys caregiver's directions. Usually follows rules at house.
Elementary school	Often violates school rules; often acts before thinking. Often engages in dishonest behavior.	Usually follows rules at school; can think before acting. Has developed an internal code of honest conduct.
Adolescence	Often violates societal rules. Unaware of own behavior and its impact on others.	Usually follows rules of society. Aware of own behavior and its impact on others.

Child Social Development: Bonding with others and learning social skills

Age	Struggling child	Successful child
Infant/toddler	Insecure attachment or bond with parent.	Secure attachment or bond with parent.
Preschool	Mostly negative interactions with parents and peers. Poor social skills.	Mostly positive interactions with parents and peers. Good social skills.
Elementary school	Mostly negative interactions or withdrawn with peers and teachers. Often affiliates with negative peers. Ineffective in solving social problems.	Mostly positive interactions with peers and teachers. Affiliates with positive peers. Solves social problems effectively.
Adolescence	Often engages in negative activities with peers or is withdrawn. Rejects family and has poor family relationships.	Engages in positive activities with peers. "Launches" from family but maintains strong family ties.

Child Emotional Development: Learning to understand/express feelings, think rational or helpful thoughts, and regulate stress-related emotions

Age	Struggling child	Successful child
Infant/toddler	Displays mostly negative basic emotions. Expresses negative emotions through play.	Displays all basic emotions. Expresses a wide range of emotions through play.

Age	Struggling child	Successful child
Preschool	Verbally unexpressive and keeps feelings inside.	Verbally expresses simple emotions.
Elementary school	Fears persist. Doesn't understand, express, and control intense emotions. Mostly negative and unhelpful thoughts about self and others.	Overcomes most fears. Understands, expresses, and controls intense emotions. Mostly positive and helpful thoughts about self and others.
Adolescence	Negative and unhealthy identity emerging. Often depressed, anxious, or angry.	Positive and healthy identity emerging. Often happy and satisfied.

Child Academic Development: Learning self-directed academic behaviors and pursuing educational opportunities

Age	Struggling child	Successful child
Infant/toddler	Apprehensive about environment. Avoids new situations.	Explores environment. Is curious and inquisitive.
Preschool	Engages in excessive television and video games versus looking at books. Poor adjustment to school setting. Indifferent about learning.	Enjoys looking at books. Good adjustment to school setting. Excited about learning.
Elementary school	Inattentive, off-task, doesn't complete tasks. Can't manage time, organize, and plan to get schoolwork done.	Concentrates, stays on task, gets tasks done. Can manage time, organize, and plan to get schoolwork done.
Adolescence	No particular special skills or interests. No viable vocational or career plans.	Consolidating special skills and interests. Engaging in vocational or career planning and preparation.

Because children don't grow up in a vacuum, it's important to take into account how the parent and family contribute to a child's development. In this book the well-being of the parent and family are considered so that the plan can also address any stress-related problems within the family that might influence the child. Therefore, you need to know if you as a parent or your family as a unit is meeting the challenges of everyday family life. Are you **stressed** or **coping**? See the *Parent and Family Well-Being* chart to get a better idea.

Parent and Family Well-Being

Parent Well-Being: Personal functioning of parent(s)

Stressed parent	Coping parent
Overwhelmed by everyday challenges and problems.	Managing everyday challenges and problems.
Marriage or intimate partner relationship problems.	Satisfactory marriage or intimate partner relationship.
Overwhelmed by parenting responsibilities.	Keeping up with parenting responsibilities.
Limited family or friend support system.	Supportive family and/or friends.

Family Well-Being: Functioning of family relationships

Stressed family	Coping family
Distant parent–child relationship.	Close parent–child relationship.
Lack of routines and/or rituals.	Predictable routines and rituals.
Mostly negative (coercive) parent–child interactions.	Mostly positive parent–child interactions.
Mostly negative family communication and inability to resolve conflict.	Mostly positive family communication and ability to resolve conflict.

Knowing the Power of Protective Factors

Many parents wonder what causes developmental struggles in a child and whether anything can be done to make things better. A combination of genetic vulnerabilities and environmental stresses causes a child's psychological developmental struggles. As a result of genetic and environmental influences, the central nervous system of a struggling child may be different from that of a successful child.

Fortunately the effects of genetic vulnerabilities and environmental stresses are not etched in stone. **Protective factors,** such as those listed in the chart on page 19, can shield the child from genetic or environmental risks. In other words, these protective factors can increase the odds that an at-risk child can still be successful. The greater the number of protective factors, the greater the chance that the child will reclaim normal development.

Protective Factors That Influence a Child's Development

Area of influence	Specific protective factors associated with successful development
Child	Behavioral and emotional regulation skills Social skills Intellectual ability Academic skills and success Positive self-perception and self-efficacy Faith, hope, and a sense of meaning in life
Parent/family	Close relationship with a stable adult Supportive and authoritative parenting Family with predictable routines and rituals Positive parent–child interactions Positive and stable family environment
Peer	Accepted by children who have positive influence Associations with children who have positive influence
Contextual	Attends and is bonded to school Lives in safe and organized neighborhoods Opportunities for school, religious, and community activities that have positive influence

Skills-building strategies can help a child get along better in everyday life and can boost protective factors. Many of the protective factors listed in the chart are essentially skills (e.g., behavioral and emotional regulation skills) or can be the by-products of the success that comes with having such skills (e.g., positive parent–child interactions). The bottom line is that a skills-building approach can enable a struggling child to make progress and succeed. There is room for optimism and hope if you take effective action by helping your child build developmental skills!

What Is the Next Step?

Having read this chapter, you should now have a better understanding of your struggling child. For whatever reason, your child may be behind in skills development and is now struggling. Most children learn developmental skills implicitly through everyday interactions with parents and others. **But a child who is behind needs to**

have those developmental skills taught explicitly. A child can be taught skills to help him or her shift from struggling to successful. In addition, parents and family members can be taught skills to help them move from stressed to coping. In this process protective factors will gain a boost that will keep your child and family on track. The next chapter will guide you in creating a skills-building plan of action for your child and family.

2

Getting Back on Track

Coming Up with a Skills-Building Plan
for Your Child and Family

In Chapter 1, I propose taking the view that a struggling child has gotten off the developmental track. The good news is that the child can get back on course with a skills-building approach. In this chapter you'll have the opportunity to identify specific parenting strategies that will build the skills that your child and family need. It's time to come up with a plan and then get going!

Examining How Child and Family Are Doing

Let's take a closer look at your child's developmental struggles and/or the parent/family concerns that you started to familiarize yourself with in Chapter 1. Use the ***Examining How Your Child and Family Are Doing*** chart (at the end of this chapter) to rate your child, self, and family. If you are working with a practitioner, he or she can give you a valuable perspective here and help ensure that you are focusing on the most important areas.

Selecting Skills-Building Strategies to Strengthen

The next step is to identify the areas you rated a *1, 2,* or *3*: These are the areas that you will target in your skills building with your child. The skills-building chapters in this book (Chapters 4–20) are divided into six sections that correspond respectively to the four areas of child development and the two areas of parent/family well-being.

The chapter summaries that follow will help you zero in on which individual chapters might help you work on the broader areas of concern that you rated as *1, 2,* or *3.* Keep in mind that the information in each chapter of this book can be applied broadly to children in the 5- to 17-year-old age range, but there are tips on tailoring the strategies for a younger child, an older child, or a teen.

You may not be entirely sure of which chapters to tackle first. Use your best judgment and choose those areas and chapters that seem to match your goals for your child and family. Your practitioner can help you think this through. It could be that several areas and corresponding chapters appear to be useful. You cannot do everything, however, so you need to focus and select one strategy to begin with. Figuring out what to work on is a very important step.

Enhancing Your Child's Behavioral Development

Chapters 4–7 contain ideas and strategies for dealing with misbehaviors. You will learn techniques for building the parent–child bond and "managing" a child. This cluster of chapters is often the best place to begin for a child rated as struggling in behavior development.

Chapter 4. Doing What You're Told: Teaching Your Child to Comply with Parental Directives

These strategies can be used to teach your child to comply with reasonable directives and to avoid related parent–child power struggles. In this chapter you are taught how to give an effective command, to give an effective warning using an "if–then" statement, and to follow through by putting a child in time-out (preschool or elementary age) or by taking away an age-adjusted privilege (all ages). Chapter 7 is often used in conjunction with Chapter 4.

Chapter 5. Doing What's Expected: Teaching Your Child to Follow Rules

Procedures are presented for clearly stating house rules to your child and for making sure those rules are followed. There are also suggestions for stating and following through with situational rules that pertain to a particular event or place away from home, such as in a restaurant or at a relative's home. Chapter 7 is often used in conjunction with Chapter 5.

Chapter 6. Doing the Right Thing: Teaching Your Child
to Behave Honestly

Ideas for quelling dishonest behaviors such as lying, sneaking, cheating, or stealing, and for promoting honesty, are provided in this chapter. Different methods
are presented for a child whose dishonesty is impulsive, for one whose dishonesty
is related to the influence of peers, and for one who seems to view dishonesty as an
acceptable way to get what he or she wants. Chapter 7 is often used in conjunction
with Chapter 6.

Chapter 7. Staying Cool under Fire: Managing Your Child's Protesting
of Discipline and Preventing Angry Outbursts

This chapter provides information and techniques that can help you deal effectively
with your child's protests (whining, tantrums, talking back, refusing to go in time-
out or give up a privilege, and so on) when you are disciplining for misbehavior (defiance, rule breaking, or dishonesty). Procedures for preventing angry outbursts from
your child, such as routines, rules, and redirection, are also described.

Enhancing Your Child's Social Development

These chapters provide ideas and strategies for enhancing your child's social competence. You will learn methods for targeting, teaching, and guiding your child to use
social skills and for assisting the child in coping with challenging social situations.

Chapter 8. Making Friends: Teaching Your Child Social Behavior Skills

Suggestions are given for teaching and coaching your child in the development of
positive social behavior skills. This includes identifying social behaviors to work on
(e.g., sharing or negotiating), as well as teaching and coaching the social behavior(s)
with your child.

Chapter 9. Keeping Friends: Teaching Your Child Social
Problem-Solving Skills

In this chapter you are told how to teach your child to recognize when a social problem exists and how to use a step-by-step process to solve that problem. This includes

discussing and practicing social problem-solving skills with your child and using social problem solving to help siblings resolve conflict (if applicable).

Chapter 10. That Hurts!: Helping Your Child with Bullies

You can assist your child with the situation if he or she is bullied. First you are encouraged to take steps to organize adults (e.g., parents, teachers, neighbors) to be observant, coordinate with each other, and intervene whenever a bully's behavior is directed toward your child. You also are given ideas on how to teach and coach your child to ignore and/or be assertive him- or herself.

Chapter 11. Hanging with the "Right Crowd": Influencing Your Child's Peer Relationships

This chapter focuses on what you can do to reduce negative peer influences on your child while increasing positive peer relationships. Specific techniques to monitor and supervise your child's peer-related activities are noted. You are also taught how to teach and coach your child in peer-coping skills. With your support, your child can learn how to identify and avoid certain situations with peers, as well as to be assertive in handling peer pressure.

Enhancing Your Child's Emotional Development

The strategies in these chapters can be especially important for a child who is prone to worry, sadness, and/or anger. You will learn to teach your child to deal with and manage feelings better so that the feelings don't manage the child. These chapters take a lot of work and call for your child to be fairly motivated (see Chapter 3).

Chapter 12. Let It Out!: Teaching Your Child to Understand and Express Feelings

You are informed how to teach your child to identify and express feelings in a healthy way in this chapter. This is accomplished by reviewing charts to increase your child's vocabulary of feeling-related words, as well as to help your child understand how feelings affect thoughts and behavior. You also learn to teach and coach your child to express feelings verbally.

Chapter 13. You Are What You Think: Teaching Your Child to Think Helpful Thoughts

Strategies in this chapter can be used to assist your child in thinking helpful thoughts. There are ideas for explaining the connection between thoughts, feelings, and behavior so that your child is more aware of how one impacts the others, and vice versa. There are also suggested ways to teach and coach your child to recognize unhelpful thoughts and replace them with helpful thoughts.

Chapter 14. Stress Busters: Teaching Your Child to Manage Stress

Procedures to help your child learn skills for managing stress are described in this chapter. You are encouraged to assist your child in developing *stress-prevention habits* like exercise, eating healthy food, getting sufficient sleep, socializing more, etc. Then you are guided to teach and coach your child in practicing *stress-coping skills* to manage high-stress episodes, including recognizing stress signals, employing relaxation techniques and calming self-talk, and taking action.

Enhancing Your Child's Academic Development

Chapters in this section give parents ideas and strategies that directly and indirectly promote children's academic success. The focus is not on teaching specific academic abilities per se (like reading or math). Instead the goal is to promote skills that facilitate academic success and to work with the school to provide what your child needs.

Chapter 15. Surviving School: Teaching Your Child to Manage Time, Organize, Plan, Review, and Stay on Task

This chapter offers many ideas for teaching your child "school survival skills." You are advised to set up a consistent time for homework each school night. This routine can be used as a platform for getting homework done and for teaching and coaching organizing, planning, and reviewing skills.

Chapter 16. Teaming Up: Collaborating and Advocating for Your Child at School

You can influence your child's school behavior and academic progress by working effectively with school officials. This chapter gives you ideas for the best ways to collaborate with school officials and to advocate for your child to receive needed services at school.

Enhancing Your Well-Being as a Parent

The focus of these chapters is on your own personal functioning. The theme is that your doing well helps your child do better too. You learn to change unhelpful thoughts and cope with stress, both of which can improve your parenting and in turn help your child.

Chapter 17. You Parent the Way You Think: Thinking Helpful Thoughts to Enhance Parenting

In this chapter you are made more aware of parenting-related thoughts. There are also instructions for restructuring unhelpful "parent thoughts" to make them more helpful. In addition, the point is made that you must stay calm to think straight when interacting with your child.

Chapter 18. Cool Parents: Managing Your Own Stress to Enhance Parenting

There are many ways you can manage stress and stay calm. In so doing, you will be more effective in parenting. In this chapter you are counseled to make stress-reducing lifestyle changes and to "be mindful" while parenting. You are also taught steps for staying calm when highly stressed out by your child in the moment.

Enhancing Your Family's Well-Being

Of course, the family's well-being can have a powerful effect on whether a child struggles or succeeds. The chapters in this section pertain to how the family unit is doing. Parents will learn methods to enhance broader family relationships and interactions.

Chapter 19. Let's Get Together: Strengthening Family Bonds and Organization

This chapter provides ideas for building parent–child bonds through activities, enhancing family connections via rituals, and improving family organization through routines. Many commonsense ideas are presented to get your family working together again.

Chapter 20. We Can Work It Out: Strengthening Family Interaction Skills

This chapter gives you strategies to improve day-to-day family interactions. You'll learn how to guide your family to use effective communication, problem-solving, and conflict management skills. These skills are important at any age but especially as a child moves into the preteen and teen years.

Figuring Out Where to Start and Getting Others' Input

The *Selecting Skills-Building Strategies to Work On* form (at the end of this chapter) can help you prioritize your focus and efforts. This chart can also be used to get input from other family members. This is a particularly good place to make decisions collaboratively with your practitioner, who will be able to call on a wealth of experience regarding what works best in certain circumstances. Put a checkmark next to the chapters that seem to apply to the needs of your family.

Understanding the Skills-Building Method

Now that you have identified areas of focus and selected corresponding skills-building chapters, you're almost ready to begin the work. But first I'd like to arm you with some principles that, if followed faithfully, will enhance your chances of success with the intervention you've started to design. The rest of the book will apply these principles within each chapter.

The "P's to Success" for Developing New Skills

According to the research, the skills-building strategies described in this book work—with one catch: They have to be implemented well! No doubt you've heard of the "keys to success." This phrase generally describes what one must do to succeed in some sort of undertaking. In this book we are going to rely on the four "P's to success." The P's help organize your efforts for achieving goals related to skills building. I strongly recommend that you use these P's to success with the chapters and skills you have chosen.

Preparing is an essential first step for putting a skills-building strategy into action. It is vital that you really know, understand, and plan how to use all of the procedures for a chosen strategy. Read and review the chapter describing it very carefully. Discuss it with your family's practitioner. Test yourself on the information by explaining it to someone. Make sure that you and your parenting partner (if applicable) understand all the information in the selected chapter. Keep studying it until you have it nearly memorized. Come up with a plan for how you will implement the skills-building strategy, such as how you'll introduce it to your child, when you'll practice, where you'll use it, and how you'll reward your child.

Practicing is essential to ingrain the skills. Practicing skills is accomplished through role playing. This is similar to acting out a play in which the skills-building strategy is rehearsed. Numerous role-playing suggestions appear throughout the chapters in this book. Some parents feel self-conscious and uncertain about using role playing, but I hope you will try the suggestions and then stick with the practice, because it really can make a difference to do this kind of rehearsing. It helps you get used to new ways of interacting with your child that may feel awkward and therefore might be avoided without prior practice. It can help you spot stumbling blocks and points where a strategy really needs to be tweaked to work for your unique family. Your practitioner will usually encourage you to use role plays during training sessions so that you can get comfortable with the process, and the practitioner can help you over rough spots or places where you're "flubbing your lines" in a way that would compromise the whole strategy.

Progress monitoring is critical to achieving lasting success. For example, dieters who set calorie intake and weight goals and keep track of what they eat and their weight over time are more likely to lose weight than those who do not. Likewise, research says (and I know from 20-plus years of working with families) that those who set goals and monitor their progress do better than those who do not. The chapters in this book provide ideas for monitoring progress related to applying the

PREPARING AND PRACTICING WITH THE HELP OF A PRACTITIONER

It can be challenging for many reasons to get going and practice new skills techniques. The preparing and practicing phases are typically best accomplished with the assistance of a practitioner. The practitioner will know how to motivate everyone and can orchestrate the skills-building effort. More often than not, you will reach your goals and see progress if you get started and continue working with a practitioner.

skills and for gauging how well your child and family are doing in day-to-day life over time. There are three types of progress monitoring: First, you will see that most of the chapters contain *Parent Checklist* forms. The checklists can be used to keep track of progress in implementing specific skills at home. Second, Chapter 3 encourages you to complete a *Parenting Goals* form and/or your child to fill out a *Personal Goals* form. The goals form can be used to set goals and measure progress that is tailored to you. You can use this for several goals that may cut across several chapters (e.g., one goal from Chapter 4 and another from Chapter 12). Third, the *Examining How Your Child and Family Are Doing* forms introduced earlier, can also be filled out later to see how much progress your child and family have made in terms of day-to-day child and family functioning.

You can use one or more of these progress monitoring methods. It is up to you to select the one that you prefer. Don't skip progress monitoring. Doing it will increase the likelihood of your child's and your family's success.

PERCONing, or implementing skills-building strategies in a **PERsistent** (over the long term) and **CONsistent** (in the same repetitive manner) manner, is fundamental to success. In other words, you have to persistently keep doing it, over weeks or months, and consistently do it in the same way (following each step, each and every time).

The Phases of Skills Building

Keep in mind that the skills-building process typically unfolds over three phases.

- First there is an **intensive phase**, often 4–8 weeks, during which you need to really concentrate and make a daily effort to practice and use the new skills, fill out charts, monitor progress, etc.

- Then there is a **maintenance phase**, typically lasting several months, during which you have to still be mindful of the new skills and keep at their application.

- Finally, there is a **relapse prevention phase,** when you and your child are using the skills naturally every day, and the goal is to keep the skills practice going over the long term and avoid slipping back.

At each phase you need to be diligent and follow through. These are not easy skills to learn and master. **More often than not, it is best to consult with your** family's practitioner to make sure you learn and apply the skills in the best way possible.

What Is the Next Step?

You should now have a plan to help your child and family, so it's time to put that plan into action. Chapter 3 will give you ideas for how to get motivated and keep going over the long haul. The rest of the book will then give you concrete ideas and strategies for accomplishing your goals. Your practitioner can assist you all the way.

Examining How Your Child and Family Are Doing

Name: _____ Date: _____

Read the descriptors from left to right that correspond to **areas of child functioning** and **areas of parent/family functioning**. Circle a number from 1 to 6 to reflect your best judgment. Underline specific words that best describe your child. *The first time you fill this out, think about your child/family in a general sense; other times you fill it out, think about your child/family over the past week or so to give you an idea of progress.* Any area rated as a 1, 2, or 3 indicates a concern, and any rating of 4, 5, or 6 indicates that things are moving in the right direction.

Areas of Child Functioning

Struggling ————————→ **In Progress** ————————→ **Successful**

Defiant, doesn't follow rules, or lies, sneaks, or steals and can get upset when disciplined		*Child behavioral development*		Follows reasonable directions and rules from adults and is trustworthy and honest	
1	**2**	**3**	**4**	**5**	**6**
Aggressive, withdrawn, bothersome, or rejected (by peers and/or siblings)		*Child social development*		Bonded with others, has good social skills, and affiliates with peers who have a positive influence	
1	**2**	**3**	**4**	**5**	**6**
Keeps feelings inside, thinks unhelpful thoughts, or is stressed out, angry, or anxious		*Child emotional development*		Understands, expresses, and controls strong feelings	
1	**2**	**3**	**4**	**5**	**6**
Dislikes school, is achieving below potential, or has trouble completing school work		*Child academic development*		Satisfactorily completes schoolwork and is pursuing educational opportunities	
1	**2**	**3**	**4**	**5**	**6**

Areas of Parent/Family Functioning

Stressed ————————→ **In Progress** ————————→ **Coping**

Feels overwhelmed, has adult relationship problems, has difficulty fulfilling parenting responsibilities, or has limited support of family/friends		*Parent well-being*		Managing personal, adult relationship and parenting challenges and has supportive family/friends	
1	**2**	**3**	**4**	**5**	**6**
Distant parent–child relationships, negative parent–child interactions, or problems with family communication and conflicts		*Family well-being*		Close and positive parent–child relationships, and family members get along with each other most of the time	
1	**2**	**3**	**4**	**5**	**6**

Selecting Skills-Building Strategies to Work On

Name: _____ Date: _____

Select child and parent/family skills-building chapters from this menu that are related to ratings of 3 or lower in the same areas on the ***Examining How Your Child and Family Are Doing*** form. Put a checkmark next to the selected chapters below. **Use your judgment and choose those chapters that seem to match your goals for your child and family.**

Enhancing Your Child's Behavioral Development

CHAPTER

____ 4. Doing What You're Told: Teaching Your Child to Comply with Parental Directives
____ 5. Doing What's Expected: Teaching Your Child to Follow Rules
____ 6. Doing the Right Thing: Teaching Your Child to Behave Honestly
____ 7. Staying Cool under Fire: Managing Your Child's Protesting of Discipline and Preventing Angry Outbursts

Enhancing Your Child's Social Development

CHAPTER

____ 8. Making Friends: Teaching Your Child Social Behavior Skills
____ 9. Keeping Friends: Teaching Your Child Social Problem-Solving Skills
____ 10. That Hurts!: Helping Your Child with Bullies
____ 11. Hanging with the "Right Crowd": Influencing Your Child's Peer Relationships

Enhancing Your Child's Emotional Development

CHAPTER

____ 12. Let It Out!: Teaching Your Child to Understand and Express Feelings
____ 13. You Are What You Think: Teaching Your Child to Think Helpful Thoughts
____ 14. Stress Busters: Teaching Your Child to Manage Stress

Enhancing Your Child's Academic Development

CHAPTER

____ 15. Surviving School: Teaching Your Child to Manage Time, Organize, Plan, Review, and Stay on Task
____ 16. Teaming Up: Collaborating and Advocating for Your Child at School

Enhancing Your Well-Being as a Parent

CHAPTER

____ 17. You Parent the Way You Think: Thinking Helpful Thoughts to Enhance Parenting
____ 18. Cool Parents: Managing Your Own Stress to Enhance Parenting

Enhancing Your Family's Well-Being

CHAPTER

____ 19. Let's Get Together: Strengthening Family Bonds and Organization
____ 20. We Can Work It Out: Strengthening Family Interaction Skills

3

Taking Care of Business
Getting Going and Following Through

The skills-building strategies in this book won't work unless you (and your child) are focused, work hard, and then follow through. This is, of course, easier said than done. Anyone who has tried to change his or her behavior, like following through with a new diet and exercise program, knows how hard it is to actually do it!

To take care of business you need to set goals, have a "can-do" attitude, and keep track of your progress until you achieve success. **Setting goals** has to do with explicitly defining what you want to accomplish. **Getting motivated** involves mustering up the desire and confidence to work hard toward achieving your goals. Finally, **monitoring progress** pertains to keeping track of how you are doing until you reach your goals. This chapter will give you ideas for taking care of business as it relates to the hard work of learning and using new skills and guiding your child similarly.

This may well be the most important chapter in this book because it centers on the key ingredients needed to effectively execute the plan you came up with in Chapter 2. If you use the methods described in this chapter, you will be on course to succeed. One thing to keep in mind, however, is that you do not need to use all of the strategies described in this chapter. It would be too much work to do so anyway! Rather, as you read this chapter, think about which methods sound like they might be helpful for you and your child, and then try one or two of them. Your family's practitioner can also provide valuable assistance in determining how to take care of business.

Choosing a Focus for Getting Going and Following Through

The *Parent Checklist for Getting Going and Following Through* (at the end of this chapter) will give you an idea of steps you can take to facilitate the work of learning and actually using new skills. This checklist also provides an overview of what this chapter is about. It is a good idea to begin by pinpointing where you and your child are now and focus on what needs to get going and what you need to follow through on. Later, if you begin to backslide, you can refer to the same checklist as a reminder of what to do to get reenergized and back on track.

Considering the Stages of Change

Knowing how ready, willing, and able different family members are will help you determine where to begin in the skills-building process. There are five stages of change that people typically go through as they work toward accomplishing challenging goals:

1. **Precontemplation.** This is where someone is not too aware of a problem or may be just entertaining the notion of making a change or working on a goal. For example, you might think "Maybe my son [or daughter] could use some assistance with making friends" or "Perhaps our family should try to get along better." A child might think "I wish I had more friends" or "Our family is messed up!"

2. **Contemplation.** This is the stage when someone is beginning to think that a plan for change is needed. For example, you might think "I should teach him [or her] some social skills" or "Our family should work on communicating better." A child might think "Maybe I should try to get along better with others" or "We need to communicate better."

3. **Preparation.** This is the stage when someone is coming up with a plan of action and goals have been set. For example, you might look at Chapter 8 to get ideas about teaching a child social skills and set a goal to work on a specific social behavior. Another parent might look at Chapter 20 and determine that family members will work on specific communication skills. A child might agree to work on cooperating and expressing feelings to others or setting a personal family communication goal of listening to others.

4. **Action.** At this point you are implementing a plan and working on goals. Either you or your child, or both of you, have been making changes in behavior for a few weeks or months and are dealing with setbacks if they occur. For example, you might teach expressing feelings and monitor your son's (or daughter's) progress using the *Feelings Diary* form (at the end of Chapter 12)

or set some communication goals and evaluate the family's progress using brief family meetings to review the *My Family Communication Goals* form (at the end of Chapter 20). A child might make an effort to work on social skills related to cooperating with others and expressing feelings or make an effort to listen to other family members.

5. **Maintenance.** You are now upholding the changes made and the new behaviors that have become routine and long-lasting. These changes have been maintained with few setbacks for a few months. For example, you have regularly coached a son or daughter in social skills so your child can maintain progress with friends. Or you have led family members to agree that when any of you slip up, you can give each other feedback about your communication. A child might show that getting along with others or communicating effectively with other family members is becoming second nature.

It can be helpful to know where all family members are in the stages of change. Filling out the *Determining Stages of Change* form (at the end of this chapter) will help you figure out what stage each family member is at so you can plan accordingly.

- **If either you or your child is at Stage 1 or 2,** it would be wise to emphasize the sections below about setting goals and getting motivated.

- **If you and/or your child is at Stage 3, 4, or 5,** you could put most of your effort into learning and using the skills described in Chapters 4–20 and focus on the sections having to do with setting goals and monitoring progress. But it still could be useful to review the sections on getting motivated for someone at Stage 3 or 4. Use your judgment or seek the input of a practitioner.

It's not unusual for a parent and child to be at different stages. And sometimes the whole family has trouble getting past Stage 1, 2, or 3. This is also where working with a practitioner can be very helpful.

Setting Parenting Goals, Getting Motivated, and Monitoring Progress

The steps in this section will help you put the plan into action by setting some concrete goals, prioritizing how important those goals are, pledging how much effort you are willing to commit, and keeping track of your progress.

Setting Parenting Goals and Getting Motivated

In Chapter 2 you selected the child and family skills-building strategies you want to work on, and now it is a good idea to set one or more related specific parenting goals. Be sure to identify specific target areas that you want to work on and related skills-training strategies. For example, you may be concerned about your child's defiance and angry outbursts whenever you attempt to discipline him or her. In this case you might set parenting goals to use a time-out and a patient standoff strategy (see Chapters 4 and 7). Another example: You and your child have ongoing conflict over homework and you are concerned that your daily family routine is unpredictable, so you set parenting goals to use a mandatory homework procedure and other daily routines to make family life more organized (see Chapters 15 and 19). **Whenever possible, try to verbalize parenting goals as *specific dos*, like "Give effective commands" or "Firmly enforce bedtime," and not *vague don'ts*, like "Stop nagging him [son] to comply" or "Don't be so disorganized."** It will help if you write down your parenting goals and review them with your practitioner.

How important are these parenting goals to you? You probably have a million things to do that relate to work, household chores, taking care of the family, and more. Plus every now and then you might want to take a break or do something enjoyable! Determining how important a chosen skills-related parenting goal is compared to all of your other obligations and interests will help you be realistic at the outset and then stay on track. Use the following scale to rate how important working on the chosen goal is in relation to all of the other things in your busy life.

Importance of Selected Parenting Goals

1	2	3	4	5	6	7	8	9	10

Not important   Somewhat important   Very important

It may be helpful to do some more thinking if your priority score is 7 or below. Examine the pros (benefits) and cons (challenges) for the parenting goal(s) you chose. Typically the pros are that the child and family might make progress, and the cons are that it is a lot of work and you may have to put less emphasis on other work, family, and recreational activities for a while. Figure out which is greater—the pros or the cons. If the pros outweigh the cons, then perhaps you should treat your parenting goals as a higher priority. If there are two or more parenting partners, and you disagree about priorities, you'll have to discuss your differences and resolve them before moving forward. This may involve compromise, and if you can't reach it on your own, a practitioner should be able to assist. Eventually you have to settle on one or two child and/or family skill areas and prioritize your parenting goals and effort accordingly. It is best to work on parenting goals or strategies that are sincerely prioritized as an 8 or higher.

Like anything in life worth achieving, you're going to have to invest hard work in building skills with and for your child. To sustain the hard work involved, you need to be committed. Pledging how much effort you intend to put into reaching your parenting goals establishes your commitment and "keeps you honest." Use the following scale to decide on and record your level of commitment.

Effort Pledge for Working on Parenting Goals

1   2   3   4   5   6   7   8   9   10

Little effort   Okay effort   Lots of effort

Did you rate your commitment at an 8 or higher? You won't get too far unless you can honestly and wholeheartedly commit maximum effort to the cause. Then you need to hold yourself accountable and put in the effort you pledged to reach your parenting goals.

Monitoring Progress on Parenting Goals

You can informally work on parenting goals in the coming days and weeks. This is the most convenient way but not necessarily the best way to work on goals (the best ways are discussed next). The informal method involves verbally stating your parenting goals and perhaps writing them down. Then periodically check in with yourself, your parenting partner (if applicable), and/or your practitioner about how it is going. Maybe schedule on the calendar that you will take stock every other day for a few weeks and later once a week after some progress has been made. Be sure to think of examples of when you did or did not work on your parenting goals (but could have worked on them). Try to be aware of your parenting goals on a day-to-day basis.

The *Parenting Goals* form (at the end of this chapter) can be used to more formally declare specific parenting-related goals and track your progress. You can customize your own parenting goals and keep track of your progress by using this form. For example, after reading Chapter 8, a mother chose to work on her child's social behaviors as an area of focus. Then she set a parenting goal of "Help my child learn and use social skills of sharing and cooperating in play." Steps to accomplish this might be "Do two brief role plays per day for 1 week," "Conduct a 10-minute family meeting once a day for 2 weeks to review progress," "Remind [child] to share and cooperate when playing with his sister or friends," etc. Another example is a father who decided that family interactions were a primary concern and then read Chapter 20. He indicated this goal on the *Parenting Goals* form: "We will work on communications skills." Steps to accomplish this might include "Ask family members to set personal communication goals," "Organize and lead 10-minute family meetings on Monday and Thursday evenings for the next 3 weeks to review communications skills (write it on calendar)," and "Make brief statements so my children listen better."

You can set similar goals based on the areas you think are important and with regard to the corresponding chapters you read. Later you can also refer to the *Parenting Goals* form occasionally until you reach your goals. You can focus on one skill or goal within a chapter or multiple skills or goals across chapters using the *Parenting Goals* form. The form can be filled out and just looked at now and then to gauge progress, or copies could be made and filled out periodically to track progress.

You will note that the *Parenting Goals* form uses a 1–3 scoring format for gauging progress. There is no right or wrong way to fill out the form. It is your own personalized way to evaluate your progress toward meeting your parenting goals. At the beginning it is a good idea to evaluate where you are in relation to a goal or step to show where you started. Thereafter, periodically revisit the *Parenting Goals* form to assess progress via the 1–3 rating. You should also think about how often and when to do the evaluation on the *Parenting Goals* form. The intervals are strictly up to you; it's just a good idea to have a plan. Consider the goal or step achieved whenever you are satisfied, usually after several days or weeks of 3 ratings. Although this process is about setting your own parenting goals and monitoring your own progress, it can be helpful to do this with a practitioner, who can also give you additional ideas.

Another way to track progress formally is by periodically reviewing the *Parent Checklist* forms that are in nearly all of the chapters of this book. The *Parent Checklist* forms provide a brief review of each skill and subskill in that chapter. You can review a form now and then to measure progress on skills acquisition. You will know that you have really learned the skill(s) whenever you consistently rate yourself as a 3 on the different skills depicted on the various *Parent Checklist* forms.

Assisting Your Child in Setting Personal Goals, Getting Motivated, and Monitoring Progress

Let's face it. It is quite possible that your child will not be too excited to learn new skills or change behavior! It is vital to get your child's cooperation, however, especially for the material in Chapters 8–15, which focus on the child's own personal skills development, and Chapters 19–20, which are about the family. **Getting a child on board and actually doing some skills-related work can be difficult, so it is frequently best to work on this section with the help of a practitioner.**

Promoting Parent–Child Collaboration with a Teamwork Approach

Parents are usually more motivated to learn new skills than children. A child might feel defensive, like he or she is always the focus and this is just another way to point out how "bad" he or she is. **If your child is unmotivated and/or defensive, it helps to emphasize a team approach.**

Sit down for a family meeting when everyone is calm and in a good mood to discuss working as a team. It can be very helpful to have this type of meeting with a practitioner, who can keep the meeting going in a productive direction. Broach the topic of the child's struggles. Use a supportive and empathic manner and tone to bring up the topic(s). Convey that you feel for your child and understand that things are sometimes tough for him or her. **Make it known that you want to help in a new way that emphasizes working together instead of arguing or avoiding discussion.** Ask your child to join with you as a team in figuring out a plan and in learning new ways to do things.

Be sure to communicate, through words and actions, that you are also working on skills and trying to improve. You can even use many of the same ideas and charts found in different chapters of the book yourself. Tell your child that your family will work together on goals. Each team member can assist others in learning and using new skills. For example, everyone could work on social behavior skills (Chapter 8) or stress management skills (Chapter 14) and complete some of the same forms, or perhaps a child could work on identifying and expressing feelings (Chapter 12) while a parent focuses on developing family routines (Chapter 19). By being a good role model and creating a team feeling, you will undoubtedly increase your child's cooperation and effort.

You probably know better than anyone how your child is likely to react to this discussion. On the other hand, when a family has been dealing with a child's significant problems for a long time, and a lot of conflict has arisen around these struggles, parents are sometimes overly pessimistic and anticipate greater resistance from their child than they might meet. Children who have come to expect to be chastised and asked to do things they don't have the skills to do can feel enormous relief when offered the opportunity to engage in a positive team effort. If you have any doubt that you can conduct this conversation with your child fruitfully, ask your practitioner for guidance or to facilitate the conversation. The practitioner can probably model how you might talk to your child, even giving you specific words to use that will help you demonstrate your feelings for your child and your hopes that you can accomplish something valuable to the whole family by working together.

Assisting Your Child in Setting Personal Goals and Monitoring Progress

Chapters 8–15 are focused on the child's acquisition of new skills, and your role as a parent is to guide your child through the process. **It is important that your child "buy into" this plan, cooperate, set goals, and commit to doing some work.** The "team" should select some skills that could be worked on and determine the corresponding chapter (e.g., stress management, in Chapter 14). Then it is a good idea to prompt your child to consider specific personal goals to work on (e.g., getting more sleep and learning/practicing the diaphragmatic breathing technique). Introduce the skills and personal goals and keep discussing them calmly until your child is willing to put in some effort (see the sections below on child motivation for more ideas if you get stuck).

It is important for your child to declare one or more personal goals, and you can help the child arrive at them. A younger child will probably benefit from your suggestions (e.g., "How about working on getting along better with your sister?"), whereas an older child or teen might profit from your general guidance (e.g., "What goals would you like to work on?"). It is always helpful to generate a list of possible personal goals and then select one or two to work on.

One way to work concretely on goals is to use one of the many forms provided throughout this book. For example, a child could work on expressing feelings and, with your guidance, periodically complete the *Feelings Diary* form (at the end of Chapter 12) to monitor progress. Another child could work on coping skills for stress and, again with the guidance of a parent, complete the *Staying Calm Worksheet* (at the end of Chapter 14) now and then to aid in learning and using that skill. Still another child could work on personal communication goals and, along with other family members, fill out the *My Family Communication Goals* form (at the end of Chapter 20) on occasion to monitor progress. Many other similar goal-related and monitoring-type forms are found in other chapters. All of these forms contain ideas and specific instructions for helping a child to use them.

Another option is to ask him or her to use one of the *Personal Goals* forms at the end of this chapter. This form can be used to personalize your child's goals and to work on goals that cut across chapters. With a younger child it is best to use the *Basic* form. Keep goals simple and assess progress now and then using a three-point scale. The parent can give the child feedback too. With an older child or teen the

Advanced goals form can be used to customize personal goals and to keep track of progress. Write down more specific personal goals that the older child or teen could work on. For example, goals could be to get more sleep, learn and use diaphragmatic breathing, or practice verbal expression of feelings. The form works best if you state personal goals and the small steps that will be taken to reach them. For example, under the goal of getting more sleep, a child could work on steps such as "I will follow a sleep routine on school nights," "I will be in bed with lights out by 9:00 on school nights," etc. The *Personal Goals (Advanced)* form can be referred to periodically until the goals are accomplished. Understand that **you need to be very much involved in helping your child set personal goals and assist him or her in periodically gauging progress.**

Promoting Your Child's Motivation to Work on Goals

The section above on setting and following through with personal goals will work with a motivated child. But if your child is not all that excited about working on personal goals, it can help to emphasize motivational techniques prior to, or simultaneously with, the goal-setting and monitoring strategy. Several methods for promoting internal and external motivation can be used.

A worksheet that can help an older child or teen get motivated is the *Thinking about Personal Goals* form at the end of this chapter (not for younger children). Write down a goal that you think would be good for your child to work on (e.g., getting more sleep or learning diaphragmatic breathing). Go through all of the questions and sections on the worksheet for that goal. The questions are very similar to the ideas presented earlier to get parents motivated. Keep discussing motivation until your child is willing to put in some effort on the chosen personal goal. You may need to repeat this each time a new personal goal is identified.

In a perfect world your child would "see the light," express a desire to work on goals, and be internally fired up to work on learning new skills. But that is not what typically occurs. Sometimes a child needs a "jumpstart" to get started and keep working. This jumpstart is especially useful for a younger child and/or an older child or teen who is at the precontemplation or contemplation stage of change. **Temporarily providing an opportunity to earn rewards for their effort is the jumpstart that many children need.** Some parents see this as "bribery," or as unnecessary, because the child "should be doing this already." But keep in mind that the external motivation of a reward can be a way to get your child to try something, which could lead to internal motivation once the child sees that the effort is fruitful.

Here are several pointers and some examples for selecting and using rewards:

- Make sure that your child knows exactly what to do to earn the reward (e.g., fill out five charts or worksheets to earn a specified reward).

- Make sure that any reward chosen is really motivating to your son or daughter *and* realistic for you to give.

- Rewards can be privileges that your child already has, but now you allow him or her to "earn them" (e.g., you could make video game time a reward to earn each day).

- Social and privilege rewards (e.g., time and activities with parents or friends) work better than material rewards (e.g., toys, cars, money) over the long term.

Examples of Rewards for a Younger Child

- Use of TV or computer for 2 hours during 1 day

- Take a 30-minute walk or play a favorite 30-minute game with a parent

- Special snack

- Parent cooks a favorite meal

- Have a friend over for supper

- Earn one token per day until the child collects three tokens to exchange for a movie

- Earn one token per day until the child collects five tokens to exchange for a 1-day fishing outing or sporting event with parent(s)

Examples of Rewards for an Older Child or Teen

- Some of the preceding (depending on age and the child's preferences)

- 30 minutes longer to stay out with friends on a weekend

- Earn one token per day until the child collects 10 tokens to exchange for a concert

- Extra driving privileges for a day

Remember, rewards are not meant to be offered forever! They should be faded out gradually, though exactly when is a judgment call. The general idea is to discontinue the rewards after your child develops a more positive attitude and has made some progress.

Illustrations of Getting Going and Following Through

Gail intends to work with her 8-year-old son, Ben, on developing social skills. She explains the idea to him and asks him to work with her as a team so that they can get

PROGRESS MONITORING WITH OCCASIONAL 10-MINUTE FAMILY MEETINGS

Another very helpful method and less formal way to monitor progress is to conduct occasional 10-minute family meetings at home. During those 10 minutes, review how it's going and troubleshoot any problems that are emerging in using skills-building strategies. Sometimes it is helpful to do more goal-setting and role-play practice. Keep the meetings positive, review successes more than problems, and be sure to close after 10 minutes (perhaps use a timer). It is a good idea for you to prepare ahead so you can focus on the most important topics and get your child's input for the agenda. You may want to have these meetings fairly often when you are getting started and then less frequently once you are making some progress. Siblings can be involved if you view them as part of the problem or if they are impacted by the child in some way.

along better. She wants to teach Ben several targeted social skills, as presented in Chapter 8, and she wants him to see these skills as personal goals to work on achieving. They discuss the teamwork approach and that they will work on this together. Ben eventually agrees to work on two new social behaviors (starting conversations and taking turns). He is interested in earning tokens for practicing and using social skills to earn extra privileges. They work out a deal that if he satisfactorily completes five role-play exercises and five *Personal Goals (Basic)* forms, he can earn pizza for dinner. Gail also declares a few parenting goals on the *Parenting Goals* form. She set a goal of "Help Ben learn and use social skills of starting conversations and taking turns." Steps to accomplish this might be "Make sure we do seven practice role plays," "Ask Ben to fill out five *Personal Goals (Basic)* forms in the next week," "Coach Ben to start conversations and take turns when playing with his brother or cousins."

Lakeisha, age 15, has problems with stress and anxiety. During a supportive and productive family meeting, her parents suggest that Lakeisha work on stress management skills. At first she is not too excited about this prospect, but with the parents' guidance, she completes the *Thinking about Personal Goals* form. Through this process Lakeisha eventually decides that it would be a good idea for her to work on stress management. Her parents have read Chapter 14 of this book and are knowledgeable about some of the skills involved in stress management. In the next session with their practitioner they all discuss ideas related to stress prevention and healthy habits and some of the techniques for coping with stress and staying calm in tense moments. Lakeisha is encouraged to declare several goals on the *Personal Goals (Advanced)* form related to developing better health habits, as well as coping with stress. She agrees and sets a personal goal to "Improve daily health habits." She notes several steps for reaching this goal, including "Improve sleep schedule on school nights," and "Go on bike rides a least four times a week." She sets another personal goal of "Handle stress better." She notes several steps to help her reach this goal, including "Practice breathing exercises for 5 minutes each day" and "Write down a list of coping self-statements that I can say to myself when stressed out." Finally, she also writes down a goal that she will fill out the ***Staying Calm Worksheet*** (at the end of Chapter 14) each day for a week to practice staying calm.

Finally, Rob and Gina, parents of 16-year-old Josh, have set out to improve the communication patterns in their family. They conduct several family meetings to develop a family teamwork perspective and to review family communication skills (see Chapter 20). Josh thinks it is a good idea for their family to improve on communication, but he is especially excited to earn extra privileges for practicing and using communication skills. All family members agree to complete the ***My Family Communication Goals*** form (at the end of Chapter 20) each day for a while. Josh will earn a movie with a friend after satisfactorily completing seven of the forms.

Parent Checklist for Getting Going and Following Through

Name: _____ Date: _____

In the blanks below, check off whether you have accomplished any of the indicated ideas related to getting going and following through.

Determining the Stages of Change for Family Members

A. _____ Figuring out what stage each family member is at for making changes.

1. *Precontemplation:* Who in the family is not too aware of a problem or a need to change or work on goals?

2. *Contemplation:* Who in the family is beginning to think that it might be a good idea to make some changes or work on goals?

3. *Preparation:* Who in the family is coming up with a plan for change and has goals to work on?

4. *Action:* Who in the family is implementing a plan and actively working on achieving goals?

5. *Maintenance:* Who in the family has met their goals and is upholding changes with new behaviors that have become routine and long-lasting?

Note: Family members at the precontemplation or contemplation stages may need help with setting goals and getting motivated.

Parent's Use of Strategies to Get Going and Follow Through

B. _____ Setting and writing down specific parenting goals.

C. _____ Prioritizing what to work on and determining how important a parenting goal is in comparison to all other obligations and interests.

D. _____ Pledging how much effort will be put into working on parenting goals.

E. _____ Monitoring progress until parenting goals are reached.

Parent's Use of Strategies to Help Child Get Going and Follow Through

F. _____ Promoting parent–child or family teamwork approach to working on goals.

G. _____ Assisting child in declaring one or more personal goals to work on.

H. _____ Promoting child's *internal motivation* by calmly discussing personal goals, motivation to accomplish them, and steps to reach them.

I. _____ Promoting child's *external motivation* by providing rewards for working on personal goals.

J. _____ Monitoring progress until child's personal goals are reached.

Determining Stages of Change

Name of Person or Family: _____ **Date**: _____

Identify a problem or a challenge for the child, parent, or family that might be the focus of a plan for change. Then write down which stage of change different family members are at. It may be helpful for the family to discuss it until a consensus is achieved and everyone is at least at the **Preparation** stage.

The problem and/or skills-building strategy being considered is:

_____

_____

1. Precontemplation: Not too aware of a problem or a need to change. *Family member(s) at this stage*:

_____

_____

2. Contemplation: Beginning to think that it might be a good idea to make some changes.

Family member(s) at this stage:

_____

_____

3. Preparation: Coming up with a well thought-out plan for change and setting goals.

Family member(s) at this stage:

_____

_____

4. Action: Implementing the plan and working on goals, making changes in behavior for a few weeks to a few months. An occasional setback might occur, but you don't give up!

Family member(s) at this stage:

_____

_____

5. Maintenance: Sustaining changes with new behaviors that have become routine and long-lasting. Changes have been maintained with few setbacks for a few months or more.

Family member(s) at this stage:

_____

_____

Parenting Goals

Name: _____ **Date:** _____

Write down your parenting goal(s) and smaller steps to take to reach it (them). Every now and then, record a score in the circle or square to indicate how much progress you have made on each parenting goal and its steps.

Limited progress	Some progress	A lot of progress
1	2	3

Overall progress!

◯

Goal 1: _____

Steps to achieve goal:

Progress on steps

1. _____
2. _____
3. _____
4. _____

Overall progress!

◯

Goal 2: _____

Steps to achieve goal:

Progress on steps

1. _____
2. _____
3. _____
4. _____

Overall progress!

◯

Goal 3: _____

Steps to achieve goal:

Progress on steps

1. _____
2. _____
3. _____
4. _____

I commit to working on these goals.

Parent signature: _____

Personal Goals (Basic)

Name: _____ **Date:** _____

The time period when the chart will be used: _____

Indicate below which goal(s) will be worked on. At the end of the specified time period the child and parent can rate how much progress the child has made on goal(s).

Child Evaluation

I am working on the following goal(s):

How much progress have I made on goal(s)? (Circle one.)

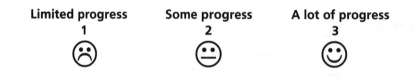

Limited progress	Some progress	A lot of progress
1	2	3

Parent Evaluation

How much progress has the child made on goal(s)? (Circle one.)

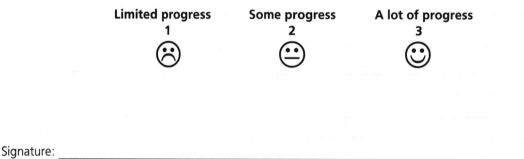

Limited progress	Some progress	A lot of progress
1	2	3

Signature: _____

Parent signature(s): _____

Personal Goals (Advanced)

Name: _____ **Date:** _____

Write down your personal goal(s) and smaller steps to take to reach it (them). Every now and then, record a score in the circle or square to indicate how much progress you have made on each personal goal and steps.

Limited progress	**Some progress**	**A lot of progress**
1	**2**	**3**

Overall progress!

Goal 1: _____ ◯

Progress on steps

Steps to achieve goal:
1. _____
2. _____
3. _____
4. _____

Overall progress!

Goal 2: _____ ◯

Progress on steps

Steps to achieve goal:
1. _____
2. _____
3. _____
4. _____

Overall progress!

Goal 3: _____ ◯

Progress on steps

Steps to achieve goal:
1. _____
2. _____
3. _____
4. _____

I commit to working on these goals and to working with my parent(s) to reach them.

Signature: _____

Parent signature(s): _____

Thinking about Personal Goals

Name: _____ **Date:** _____

It has been suggested that I work on a goal of: _____

_____

What are the "pros" or positives that might happen if I work on this goal? _____

_____

_____

What are the "cons" or negatives that might happen if I work on this goal?

_____

_____

_____

Which is greater—the *pros* or *cons* for working on this goal? (Circle one.)

How important is working on this goal compared to other activities in my life? (Circle one.)

	1	2	3	4	5	6	7	8	9	10	

Not important   Somewhat important   Very important

I agree to put in this amount of effort to work on this goal (circle one):

	1	2	3	4	5	6	7	8	9	10	

Little effort   Okay effort   Lots of effort

Rewards I might be able to earn for working on goal(s): _____

_____

I agree to work with my parent(s) on this goal.

Signature: _____

Parent signature(s): _____

Enhancing Your Child's Behavioral Development

4

Doing What You're Told

Teaching Your Child to Comply
with Parental Directives

Noncompliance occurs when a parent tells a child to do something (e.g., "Turn off the TV and come to dinner") and the child doesn't do it (e.g., keeps watching TV or doing something else). Different forms of noncompliance include **defiance,** where the child outright refuses to follow the parent's directive; **bargaining,** when the child verbally tries to strike up a deal about doing it later; and **resistance,** which occurs when the child drags it out, complains, and complies halfheartedly. Sometimes a child will **protest** by arguing, talking back, acting up, etc., when the parent tries to get the child to comply or attempts to discipline him or her for noncompliance. If your child typically displays one or more of these forms of noncompliant or

---

OVERLAPPING BEHAVIORS AND STRATEGIES

Children who exhibit high levels of noncompliance (the focus of this chapter) frequently also engage in a lot of rule-violating behavior (the focus of Chapter 5). There is an important difference between the two: Noncompliance pertains to a refusal to accede to a parent's requests (e.g., saying "No" when the parent has just told the child, "Pick up those clothes and put them in the hamper"). Rule violations involve a failure to fulfill an expectation regarding a routine (e.g., the child is rarely in bed at the prescribed time of 9:00 P.M. on school nights). Different strategies work best for each of these problem categories, but they do overlap. **Therefore it is sometimes most effective to use the skills-building strategies in both Chapters 4 and 5 at the same time.** You have to carefully consider which behaviors to target with which tactic. As a rule of thumb, it is better to target a repetitious behavior infraction (e.g., 9:00 P.M. bedtime on school nights) as a rule violation (see Chapter 5) rather than as noncompliance (e.g., every night telling the child to go to bed at 9:00 P.M.).

protesting behaviors, the ideas in this chapter may be helpful. Numerous strategies are described that can be used to get your child to comply and that can help you avoid the power struggles that often typify parent–child interactions with a noncompliant child.

Choosing a Focus for Compliance

Start by evaluating yourself on the *Parent Checklist for Child Compliance* (at the end of this chapter). This form will help you pinpoint where you are now so that you can focus effectively on what needs work. This checklist will also provide an overview of the topics covered in this chapter. You can refer to the same checklist periodically as a reminder and to measure your progress in using the new skills.

Strategy 1: Increasing Your Child's Compliance with a Positive Approach

Frequent noncompliance has a way of eroding the parent–child relationship over the years. Ongoing power struggles sometime create a wall between parent and child, and there are often more negative interactions than positive. It makes sense to begin with a positive approach: a goal of strengthening the parent–child bond and reinforcing positive behaviors in your child.

Building a Better Relationship

Building a better relationship with your child can encourage him or her to comply with your requests. Consider some of the bosses you've worked for over the years. If you liked your boss, you likely followed his or her directives and were willing to go the extra mile. If you did not exactly enjoy your boss's company, you may have put in minimal effort or even been a bit resistant at times.

The same dynamic can occur between a child and parent. As a parent you are in many ways "the boss," and your child needs to follow your directions. Your child is more likely to obey your directives if you two have a good relationship. In addition, disciplining your child for noncompliance will be more effective if you have a solid relationship foundation. For these reasons it is important to make an extra effort to establish rapport with your child and rekindle the bond between you if it has deteriorated. Try to spend more quality time together and become more involved in your child's life and activities. The "investment" in building a relationship will pay off in increasing your child's compliance. See Chapter 19 for more ideas on building the parent–child relationship.

 TROUBLESHOOTING TIP
Sometimes a child will show a lack of interest in a parent's overtures to spend time together. If this occurs, don't give up. Keep trying every now and then. In addition, many children will respond to a direct approach, such as discussing how you would like to improve your relationship, and then asking for ideas for how to accomplish this.

Avoiding Critical and Negative Comments

Dealing with a difficult child can be frustrating, and some exasperated parents can easily slip into a habit of making critical and negative comments. These types of statements do not improve behavior. It is also important to avoid saying things that can drive a wedge or create distance between you and your child, which can, in the long run, make a child's behavior worse. Try to stay away from these behaviors:

- **Criticism,** such as "You are being selfish again," "You always find a way to get out of doing your work," or "You did a good job with cleaning up today, so why can't you do that every day?"

- **Asking negative questions,** such as "Why did you do that?" or "How many times must I tell you?" or "Why do you always argue with me?"

- **Blaming,** as exemplified by "It's your fault" or "There you go again" or "You never do what I say."

- **Bringing up old issues** by saying "This is the same thing you did last week" or "Plus yesterday you . . . ," or "Last week you lied to me."

- **Putdowns,** such as "I'm sick of you," "You are such a pain in the butt," or "Are you that dumb?"

Making a conscious effort to watch what you say can go a long way toward improving the parent–child relationship. **Instead of criticizing and making negative comments, try to be direct and specific with constructive statements that**

inform your child of the specific behaviors you want or expect. Examples of these helpful statements include "Stop teasing your brother," "Let's discuss this calmly," and "Pick up the clothes on the floor now." (These kinds of effective commands are described more later in this chapter.)

Also, you don't have to agree with your child, but it is a good idea to listen to him or her and communicate that you understand his or her feelings. This type of validation can go a long way toward helping the child feel heard. This, in turn, can reduce angry acting-out episodes by your child.

Of course your child may well be saying critical or negative things to *you*. As the parent it is important for you to take the lead, set a positive example, and try to change the tone of everyday parent–child dialogue. See Chapter 20 for more ideas about facilitating effective family communication.

Catching 'Em Being Compliant

Sometimes the simplest ideas work best. If you want more compliance, it pays to notice when your child *is* compliant and reinforce it with positive attention.

Your child surely complies sometimes! Be sure to notice, comment, and praise your child for cooperating with you and/or complying with a specific request. For example:

- "Thank you, [child's name], for turning off the TV when I asked."

- "[Child's name], I liked it when you stopped bugging your brother after I told you to."

- "[Child's name], I appreciated it when you took out the garbage."

After you do this for a while, you'll be surprised by just how far some positive attention will go in improving your child's compliance. **Strive to offer at least three positive comments or praise related to your child's complying for every one correction or reprimand for noncompliance!**

 TROUBLESHOOTING TIP
Sometimes parents "forget" to notice their child's compliance. To remedy this, try pinning up a reminder note on the fridge, or ask your parenting partner (if this applies) to gently remind you, or put it in your planner/calendar to take stock and evaluate progress on catching 'em being compliant once a week (e.g., every Tuesday).

Strategy 2: Reducing Your Child's Noncompliance with a Firm Approach

Step 1: Give an Effective Command

Remember that getting your child to comply involves first telling him or her to do something. The way you tell your child to do something (i.e., *command*) is extremely important. Parents often get into the habit of using commands that don't work very well, especially for a child who is often noncompliant. Therefore it is useful to review what *not* to say for a command:

- **Vague command:** These are instructions that sound like "Knock it off" or "Shape up." They don't really say what you **do** want the child to do!

- **Question command:** These sometimes sound like "Do you want to pick up your toys?" Remember, one of the first words your child learned was *no!*

- **Rationale command:** Try not to explain to your child why a command should be obeyed, for example: "Get dressed now, because we don't have much time and I don't want us to be late." This can lead to a debate about your rationale, such as "We have plenty of time; we won't be late," and then your command gets lost in the shuffle.

- **Multiple commands:** This might be "Pick up your toys, wash your hands, come downstairs, and sit down at the table." Many children can't remember multiple commands.

- **Frequent commands:** Every parent has done this. You tell your child to do something again and again and again, while the frustration grows and grows and grows.

It's not that you should never ask your child a question or give a rationale, just not at the moment that you want compliance, especially if your child has a pattern of noncompliance. When compliance is needed, you increase the odds of your child complying if you use an **effective command:**

- Make eye contact with your child and raise your voice **slightly** (don't yell).

- Make it clear, specific, and one step.

- State the command or instruction in 10 or fewer words, such as:

- "Turn the TV off now."
- "Put your pajamas on now."
- "Pick up those toys and put them on the shelf."

- "Turn the computer off now."
- "Do your homework now."
- "Pick up your dishes from the living room."

Praise your child if he or she complies with your command, but if not, go to Step 2.

PRE-COMMANDS AND "WHEN . . . THEN" COMMANDS

Some children have a hard time transitioning from one task to another and benefit from **pre-commands,** which tell the child that compliance will soon be expected. For example, if you want your child off a computer game at 4:00, tell the child at 3:45, 3:50, and 3:55 that at 4:00 the computer must go off. Then at 4:00 give an effective command such as "Okay, it is 4:00, and I expect you to turn off the computer now."

Another useful way to get a child to comply is by using a "when . . . then" command. You tell your child that **when** he or she has completed a task, **then** he or she can have a privilege (e.g., "When you have finished with the dishes, then you can watch TV").

OCCASIONALLY NEGOTIATING AND RESTATING THE COMMAND

Now and then a parent may give a command, and then the child "bargains" by trying to strike up a deal about doing it later, doing part of it, or something similar. Technically this is a form of noncompliance. But sometimes a flexible approach is warranted, at which point it is reasonable to negotiate about the command. For example, say you tell your child, "Turn off the TV and begin your homework now." Your child then asks if he can begin homework after the show is over. If you deem this "deal" to be reasonable, you could restate the negotiated command such as "Okay, then turn off the TV and begin homework after the show." This type of collaboration can serve a benefit of avoiding power struggles and can create an atmosphere of cooperation. Use this technique sparingly, however, or it could turn into a bad habit.

Note: *The above are start commands. These are preferred because they tell a child what to do. Now and then it is okay to give stop commands such as "Stop bugging your sister." It is best to follow a stop command with a short start command (e.g., "I want you to share with your sister").*

Step 2: Give an Effective Warning Using an "If . . . Then" Statement

There are two types of warnings:

1. **Warning Linked to Time-Out (best for younger children).** Warn your child that **if** he or she doesn't (obey command), **then** he or she will be put in time-out. For example, "**If** you don't turn the video game off now, **then** you will have to go to time-out."

 TROUBLESHOOTING TIP
If you don't have time for time-out (e.g., you are getting ready for work in the morning), use privilege removal in the warning.

2. **Warning Linked to Privilege Removal (can be used with children of any age and is best for teens).** The child is told that he or she must comply or lose a privilege. **Privileges** include use of specific toys, video games, Internet, TV, cell phone, sports equipment (e.g., bicycle, basketball, hockey skates), iPod; leaving the house, hanging out with friends, using the car (if older teen), etc.

   It is a good idea to select privileges that are a "want" and not a "need." The examples above are wants for most children, but something like hanging out with friends might be a need for a socially isolated child. In that case it might be counterproductive to remove that privilege. Use your best judgment when identifying privileges that will be removed for noncompliance and take into account the want versus need idea.

Option 1: Unspecified Time Limit of Privilege Removal

Warn your child that **if** he or she doesn't (obey command), **then** he or she will lose a privilege until the child complies with the command. For example, "**If** you don't do the dishes, **then** you'll lose computer privileges until they are done."

Option 2: Specified Time Limit of Privilege Removal

The child is told that a privilege is lost **for a specified period of time** (e.g., 24 hours), and he or she is still expected to comply with the command. For example, "**If** you don't do homework now, **then** you'll lose cell phone privileges for 24 hours."

 TROUBLESHOOTING TIP
Some children will say "I don't care" in response to their parents' remov-ing a privilege. If your child says that, don't get discouraged or give up on using this idea. The child may just be trying to discourage you from following through. It is also important to have a long-term perspective with this tech-nique. Maybe your child won't care this time, but if you keep it up, day in and day out, eventually he or she will get tired of losing the privilege and will start to care. Don't give up!

Praise your child if he or she complies with your warning, but if not, go to Step 3.

Step 3: Follow Through with a Warning!

Wait a reasonable amount of time (maybe count to 5). If your child doesn't comply, then either put the child in time-out **or** take away a privilege, as warned.

Option 1: Follow Through with Time-Out for Step 3

It is a lot trickier to manage a time-out than most parents realize. Many parents enforce time-out incorrectly, and it doesn't work. Carefully study this and the "Man-aging Your Child's Protests" section below before trying time-out.

- Set up the time-out chair ahead of time. It should be located in a place where there is nothing to distract or entertain the child and where you can keep an eye on him or her. Ideally the chair would face toward a corner in a room.

- Follow Steps 1 and 2 above for an effective command and warning.

- Then put your child in the time-out chair for Step 3. If you are comfortable doing it, you can use **"physical guidance"** to bring your child to the chair. This means putting your hand on or under his or her shoulder to escort the child to time-out. **It is not a good idea to drag, push, restrain, or get physi-cally involved with your child in an attempt to put him or her in time-out.**

See "Managing Your Child's Protests" for suggestions about what to do if your child resists going to time-out.

- A general rule of thumb is 1 minute in time-out for every year of a child's age (e.g., 8 minutes for an 8-year-old).

- Use a timer! It's a helpful reminder to you and your child.

The ***Time-Out*** chart (at the end of this chapter) summarizes the procedures above. **It is a good idea to review the chart with your child and, if possible, to first do a role play in which you practice using the chart with your child as a reference so that the child knows what to expect.** Consider providing a reward to your child for doing some role playing.

TROUBLESHOOTING TIP

If using time-out, it is a good idea to require your child to comply with the original command after time-out if it is possible (e.g., the child still has to put toys on the shelf after time-out). If the child refuses again, repeat the time-out cycle.

Option 2: Follow Through with Privilege Removal for Step 3

The ***Removing Privileges for Noncompliance*** chart (at the end of this chapter) summarizes this procedure. **It is a good idea to review the chart with your child and, if possible, do a role play in which you practice using the chart as a reference so that the child knows what to expect.** Consider providing a reward to your child for doing some role playing.

TROUBLESHOOTING TIP

Sometimes when a privilege is removed for a specified time period, a child will sneak the privilege that was taken away. If you catch your child doing this, tell the child that the specified time period of that privilege loss will be restarted (e.g., start the 24 hours over).

PRACTICE EXERCISES

It is very helpful to practice Steps 1–3 to promote your child's compliance. One good place to begin is role playing a typical noncompliance situation (e.g., a child will not turn off a video game to begin the bedtime routine) and then go through the steps. Get another adult to help out and then take turns acting as the "child" and the "parent." Later you could do some role playing with your child if he or she is cooperative. You and your child can act out the steps to practice and to help your child understand what will occur at home in the future. These role plays with the child can be hard, so it may be best to do them with a practitioner's assistance.

Strategy 3: Managing Your Child's Protests of Time-Out or Removal of Privileges

It is not uncommon for a child to protest (act up) when a parent attempts to use time-out or to remove privileges in Step 3. **This protest,** which can range from sighing and groaning to talking back to throwing chairs, **is an additional target behavior on top of the noncompliance, and it warrants its own strategy.** The general idea for handling protests is to ignore them, avoid arguing, and **patiently** follow through with the time-out or privilege removal. This does not mean giving in and letting the child have his or her way. It means patiently following through without getting involved in power struggles. It also means *disengaging and deescalating* if the protesting gets out of hand (e.g., separating, avoiding verbal debates or power struggles, staying calm). **When you are targeting noncompliance using the strategies in this chapter, you may need to work on managing child protesting by using strategies in Chapter 7 at the same time.**

Achieving Success with Compliance

Compliance involves obeying and following directions given by a parent in a reasonable amount of time. This chapter provides ideas and strategies that you can use to get your child to follow reasonable parental directives. To follow through it is highly recommended that you periodically review the *Parent Checklist for Child Compliance* (at the end of this chapter) and/or set your own goals to attain with the *Parenting Goals* form (at the end of Chapter 3).

Be mindful of the fact that sometimes a child's noncompliance gets worse before it gets better once you start using these methods. Don't give up! You need to be **persistent** and **consistent** (i.e., PERCON; see Chapter 2) in applying these skills-building strategies every day until they work. Sometimes this takes weeks or months.

Parent Checklist for Child Compliance

Name: _____ **Date:** _____

In the blanks below, indicate a score for **how well** you make use of that parenting behavior at this time.

Not too well	Okay	Very well
1	2	3

Parent's Use of a Positive Approach to Increase Child's Compliance

A. _____ Building a relationship and bond

B. _____ Avoiding use of critical or negative comments

C. _____ Catching 'em being compliant by using three positive comments or praise about the child's compliance for every one correction or reprimand about child's noncompliance

Parent's Use of a Firm Approach to Reduce Child's Noncompliance

D. _____ Giving *effective commands* by making them clear, specific, one-step, and while having eye contact with the child and with voice slightly raised

E. _____ Giving *effective warnings* that *if* the command isn't followed, *then* the child will go to time-out *or* lose a privilege

F. _____ *Following through* by putting the child in time-out *or* taking away a privilege at that moment or in a delayed and patient manner if the child protests (acts up) significantly

Parent's Use of Strategies to Manage Child's Protesting of Discipline for Noncompliance

G. _____ Ignoring and not getting caught up in the child's talking back, acting up, complaining, and so on, when trying to get the child to comply (see Chapter 7 for more information)

H. _____ Disengaging from power struggles and avoiding yelling, threatening, forcing, and so on, to get the child to comply (see Chapter 7 for more information)

I. _____ Following through with D–F above in a calm manner (see Chapter 7 for more information)

Time-Out

1.
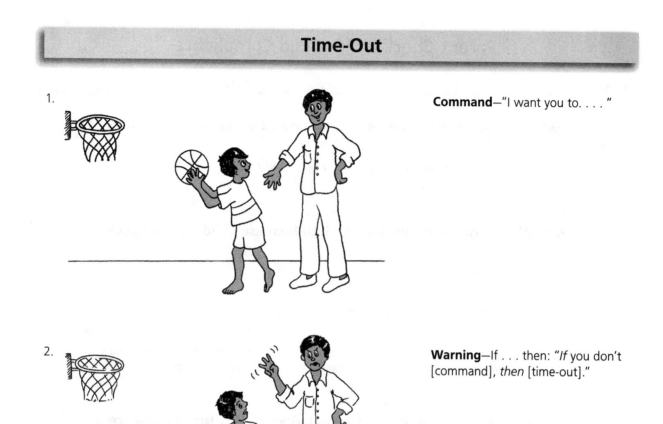

Command—"I want you to. . . . "

2.

Warning—If . . . then: "*If* you don't [command], *then* [time-out]."

3.
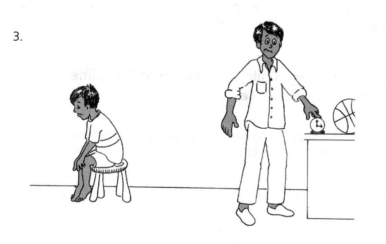

Time-out—Have the child sit and then set a timer.

Time-Out

1.

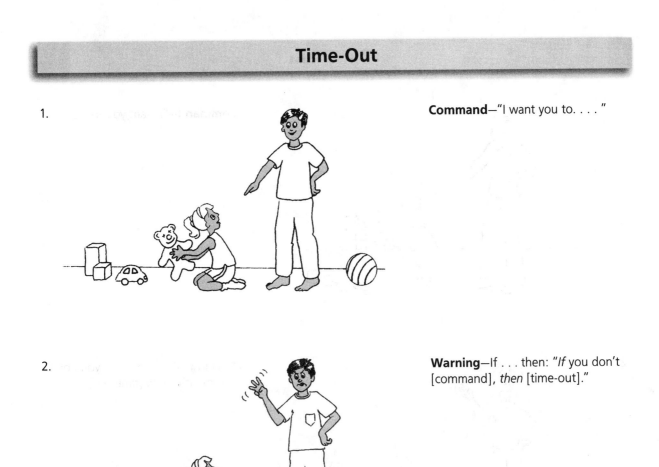

Command—"I want you to. . . . "

2.

Warning—If . . . then: "*If* you don't [command], *then* [time-out]."

3.

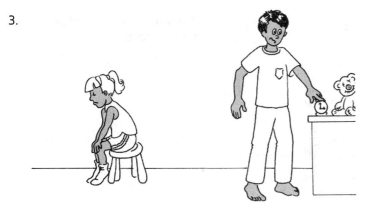

Time-out—Have the child sit and then set a timer.

1.

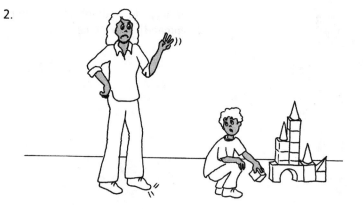

Command—"I want you to. . . . "

2.

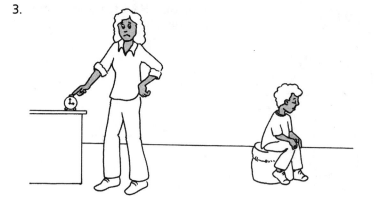

Warning—If . . . then: "*If* you don't [command], *then* [time-out]."

3.

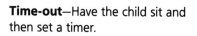

Time-out—Have the child sit and then set a timer.

Time-Out

1. **Command**—"I want you to. . . . "

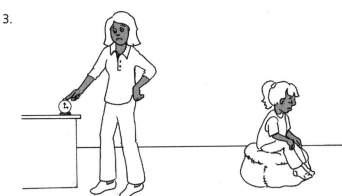

2. **Warning**—If . . . then: "*If* you don't [command], *then* [time-out]."

3. **Time-out**—Have the child sit and then set a timer.

Removing Privileges for Noncompliance

1. **Parent states a brief, clear, and specific command to child or teen.**

2. **Give a warning:** "If . . . then" statement.

   - **Option 1:** The child or teen is told *if* he or she doesn't follow command, *then* a privilege will be lost until he or she complies with the command.

   - **Option 2:** The child or teen is told *if* he or she doesn't follow command, *then* a privilege will be lost for a specified period of time (e.g., 24 hours), and he or she is still expected to comply with command.

3. **Loss of privilege.** Follow through with option 1 or 2 above.

4. Privilege return. **The lost privilege is restored in accordance with the specification of option 1 or 2 above.**

5

Doing What's Expected
Teaching Your Child to Follow Rules

Rules are behavioral expectations or codes of conduct that parents expect their child to follow without always having to be told. Many parents assume that their children understand the rules when in fact they may not. Sometimes parents have not clearly stated the rules or the child "forgets" or ignores them. Sometimes a child will protest—arguing, talking back, acting up, etc.—when the parent tries to get the child to follow rules or attempts to discipline the child for rule violations. This chapter provides ideas for clearly stating rules to your child and making sure those rules are followed.

OVERLAPPING BEHAVIORS AND STRATEGIES

Chapter 4 noted that children who exhibit high levels of noncompliance also show a lot of rule-violating behavior. **For this reason it is sometimes most effective to use the skills-building strategies in Chapters 4 and 5 at the same time. See Chapter 4 for a thorough discussion of overlapping behaviors and strategies.**

Choosing a Focus for Rule Following

Start by evaluating yourself on the *Parent Checklist for Child Rule Following* (at the end of this chapter) to help you pinpoint where you are now and focus on what needs work. This checklist will also provide an overview of the topics covered in this chapter. You can refer to the same checklist periodically as a reminder and to measure your progress.

Strategy 1: Increasing Your Child's Rule Following with a Positive Approach

Your child's rule following can be enhanced if you begin with, and intentionally focus on, a positive approach.

Building a Better Relationship and Avoiding Critical or Negative Comments

To improve rule following in your child, it is important to begin by making an extra effort to establish rapport and keep the everyday dialogue between the two of you as positive as possible. Try to spend more "quality time" together and become more involved in your child's life and activities. While you are building that relationship, make a conscious everyday effort to avoid making critical or negative comments to your child and be as constructive as possible. The investment in building a relationship and enhancing everyday discussions will pay off in increasing your child's rule-following behavior (see Chapter 4 for more details).

Catching 'Em Following Rules

Even children who frequently break rules will follow them sometimes! Be sure to notice, comment, and praise your child for following the rules. For example:

- "Thank you, [child's name], for doing your homework before 7:00."

- "[Child's name], I really liked it when you came in on time today."

- "I really appreciate it, [child's name], when you talk to your sister in a respectful manner."

Strive to offer at least three positive comments and/or praise related to your child's rule following for every correction or reprimand for rule violations!

Strategy 2: Writing Down and Discussing House Rules with Your Child

If you want your child to follow the rules and to avoid arguments about them, make sure that these rules, which we'll call **house rules,** are crystal clear. Begin this process by thinking of all the rules your child seems to violate. Often these are behaviors you frequently have to discipline or nag the child about. **Then write down the house rules on a piece of paper,** using these guidelines:

- Be very clear and specific about the rules. Instead of "Do your homework," write down "Finish your homework before 8:00 P.M. on school nights."

- Word the rules as dos rather than don'ts. This means that rules should tell the child what to do instead of what not to do. Instead of "No fighting with your brother," write down "Talk out disagreements with your brother" (if your child ends up fighting with his brother, it would still be a rule violation).

- Focus rules on important matters that are causing bigger problems (e.g., bedtime) and let the little things go that are annoying (e.g., chew food with your mouth closed).

Examples of House Rules for a Younger Child

- Complete homework by 7:00 p.m. on school nights.
- Go to bed by 8:00 P.M. on school nights.
- Be ready for the bus at 7:30 A.M. on school days.
- Make your bed before going to school.
- Brush your teeth before leaving for school.
- Feed the dog before going to school.
- Help with dishes after supper.
- Ask for permission to go anywhere outside of the yard.
- Tell a parent where you are going.
- Talk out disagreements with your brother.
- Talk to parents in a respectful manner.
- Clean up your own messes.
- Keep clothes off your bedroom floor.
- Hang up your coat and backpack.

Examples of House Rules for an Older Child or Teen

- Complete homework by 9:00 P.M. on school nights.
- Go to bed by 10:00 P.M. on school nights.
- Talk to parents in a respectful manner.
- Be in the house by 9:30 on school nights and 11:00 on weekend nights.

- Be ready to leave for school at 6:30 A.M. on school days.

- Help with dishes after supper.

- Clean up your own messes.

- Complete daily "chore list" before parent gets home from work.

- Talk out disagreements with your sister and brother.

- Call if you are going to be late.

- Limit video games to 1 hour a day.

- Make sure parents know the "4 Ws" when you are not home: <u>wh</u>ere you are, <u>wh</u>at you are doing, <u>wh</u>om you are with, and <u>wh</u>en you will be home.

Arrange your list of rules in order of importance and narrow them down. Put the most important rule at the top of the list, then the second most important, and so on. It is wise to focus on no more than four of the most important house rules at a time.

CREATE OPPORTUNITIES FOR SUCCESS WITH HOUSE RULES

It is important for your child to achieve some success with house rules or he or she will get discouraged. What's more, it might backfire if you go from having few enforced house rules to many enforced house rules. Therefore, it is a good idea to have some "easy" rules (e.g., feed the dog before going to school) along with some "hard" rules (e.g., play video games no more than 1 hour a day) so that your child can succeed. You can remove easy house rules over time and add more difficult ones later.

Then sit down with your child to discuss the house rules. **Explain that you expect your child to follow these rules.** Make sure that your child clearly understands every house rule. It may be helpful for each of you to have a written copy and/ or to post the house rules on a family bulletin board.

 TROUBLESHOOTING TIP
Sometimes a child will not cooperate with a parent's attempt to review house rules and may even become angry. If your child refuses to discuss the issue of house rules, it may be wise to tell him or her that you'll wait until another day, but that eventually you will be putting these rules into effect. If your child repeatedly refuses to discuss this issue, you will have to post the house rules without discussing them.

OCCASIONALLY NEGOTIATING AND RESTATING A HOUSE RULE

Sometimes a child will attempt to "bargain" or negotiate about a house rule. This technically may be a form of violating that rule. Now and then, however, a flexible approach is warranted, and it is then reasonable to negotiate about a house rule. For example, say that a house rule specifies a curfew time for a teen to be home on a weekend night. But the teen calls home and asks if the curfew can be extended because "the movie just got over and everyone is going to [restaurant]." If you think this "deal" is reasonable, you could restate the negotiated house rule in these terms: "Okay, just for tonight, you can come home right after you are done at [restaurant], which should be by [specified time]." This type of collaboration can serve a benefit of avoiding power struggles and can create an atmosphere of cooperation. Use this technique sparingly, however, or it could turn into a bad habit.

 TROUBLESHOOTING TIP

So far house rules have been discussed as if one set of rules applies to one child. But what if you have more than one child? One option is to have separate specific house rules for each child. This allows you to individualize house rules for each child, but it can be a lot of work. Another option is to have one set of global house rules for all children. This is more convenient but makes it hard to set specific house rules for each child. You have to weigh the pros and cons of these methods to determine which is best for you. With either approach, you would have to use the methods below for enforcing house rules on a child-by-child basis because each child will, more than likely, follow or violate house rules in his or her own way.

Strategy 3: Enforcing House Rules with Your Child

Discussing and writing down the rules, along with praising children when they follow them, may not be enough to improve some children's behavior. **If your child continues to violate the house rules generated via Strategy 2 above, you have to follow through!** There are three recommended options for following through. These options should be considered and selected based on your goals, practical matters such as how much time you have at that moment, and the age of your child. Be sure to discuss the different options with your practitioner if you are unsure which is best for your family.

Option 1: Review the House Rules Each Day to Create More Awareness

One goal of the house rules procedure is for a child to "internalize" them and to act on them automatically. This can be accomplished by reviewing the rules and asking a child to reflect on how well he or she is following them. Sit down and briefly discuss the house rules with your child on a daily basis.

- Review each house rule one at a time and ask the child to score him- or herself using the ***How Well Was I Following the House Rules Today?*** chart at the end of this chapter (e.g., the child gives him- or herself a score of *1, 2, 3,* or *4* for each house rule).

- Then you score the child for each house rule using the same chart (e.g., give the child a score of *1, 2, 3,* or *4* for each house rule).

- Discuss any differences in child and parent scores. Make sure your child understands how you came up with your score by giving examples.

- **Praise your child for scores of *3* or *4* and firmly tell him or her that scores of *1* or *2* are unacceptable.**

In addition, some children benefit from informal dialogue about the house rules throughout the day. You could remind your child of the house rules **once** (not repeatedly) as events unfold (e.g., at 8:00 you could say "Remember that one of your house rules is that you get homework done by 9:00").

Option 2: Time-Out for House Rules Violations (Usually for a Younger Child)

In Chapter 4 the time-out procedure was reviewed for use with a younger child. If you have been using time-out for your child's noncompliance, you can also use it to help the child follow rules, but with a slight difference in procedure. When promoting compliance, the procedure calls for the parent to (1) give an effective command, (2) give a warning if the child doesn't comply with the command, and (3) put the child in time-out if he or she doesn't comply with the warning.

With house rules, the written rules replace the command and warning. **Instead, you tell your child that the house rules must be followed; if they are broken, an automatic time-out results.** For example, if the house rule is "Talk out disagreements with your brother," and your child hits his or her brother, the outcome is an automatic time-out.

Option 3: Make Daily Privileges Contingent on Following House Rules

For some children it is useful to link privileges to following the house rules. These are privileges your child may already have that will now be used to motivate the child to follow house rules.

Specifying That Privileges Are to Be Earned by Following House Rules

Make sure that your child knows which privileges need to be earned. Tell your child that he or she can have access to the usual privileges if he or she follows the house rules. Examples of privileges to be earned include access to:

- Books and magazines
- Video games
- Internet
- Television
- Cell phone
- Sports equipment (e.g., bicycle, basketball, hockey skates, etc.)
- Personal music device
- Specified toys
- Going out of house
- Hanging out with friends
- Car (for older teen)

It is a good idea to select privileges that are a "want" and not a "need." The examples above are wants for most children, but something like hanging out with friends might be a need for a socially isolated child. In that case it might be counter-productive to remove that privilege. Use your best judgment—and seek your practitioner's advice—when identifying privileges that will be removed for rule violations and take into account the want versus need idea.

Stating the Time Span for Following House Rules and Access to Privileges

It is very important to specify the time span in which following house rules is linked to privileges. This time span tells the child when he or she needs to follow house rules in order to have access to certain privileges at a certain time.

With a younger child (and sometimes with an older child or teen) it is often best to link compliance with privileges earned on the same day. In other words, evening privileges (typically privileges the child can have for the last 1–2 hours before bed) are contingent on how well house rules were followed that day up to the evening. This approach has the advantage of being more immediate, but it prevents you from targeting late evening or nighttime behaviors (e.g., getting ready for, and getting into, bed).

With an older child or teen it is usually best to link compliance on one day with privileges earned on the next day. In other words, privileges for the next day (e.g., Wednesday) are contingent on how well house rules were followed that day (e.g., Tuesday). The advantage is that you can target late evening or nighttime behaviors (e.g., getting ready for, and getting into, bed), but the disadvantage is that the consequence is less immediate. Many older children and teens can usually understand and get used to the next-day method, and over time it works well. Use your best judgment—and seek your practitioner's advice—when determining whether the same-day or next-day method is best for your older child or teen.

Connecting the Following of House Rules to the Receiving of Privileges

The ***Daily Privileges for Following House Rules*** form (at the end of this chapter) can be used to help the child learn to follow house rules. To make best use of this form, first consider these guidelines:

- Specify a time period for following house rules (e.g., 6:00 A.M. to 7:00 P.M. that day if using the **same-day** method, or 6:00 A.M. that day to 6:00 A.M. the next day if using the **next-day** method).

- Write down up to four rules in the house rules column.

- Indicate privileges that can be earned or lost on the bottom of the chart according to Level A, Level B, or Level C (see examples below).

- At the end of the day, put a *Y* (yes) on the chart for house rules that were followed and an *N* (no) on the chart for house rules that were not followed (**smiling and frowning faces can be used for Y's and N's, respectively, for younger children**).

- At the end of the day, inform your child of earned privileges in accordance with how many house rules were followed.

Illustrations of Privileges for Following House Rules

- **Full privileges for following four house rules (4 Y's for Level A):** Child has privileges of video games, Internet, television, cell phone, as well as personal music device, leaving the house, hanging out with friends, books, magazines, and sports equipment that evening for the same-day method or over the next 24 hours for the next-day method.

- **Some privileges are lost for following two to three house rules (2–3 Y's for Level B):** Child has some privileges, like personal music device, leaving the house, hanging out with friends, as well as books, magazines, and sports equipment that evening for the same-day method or over the next 24 hours for the next-day method.

- **Most privileges are lost for following zero to one house rules (0–1 Y for Level C):** Child has few privileges, like only books, magazines, and sports equipment that evening for the same-day method or over the next 24 hours for the next-day method.

TROUBLESHOOTING TIP

Sometimes a child will sneak a privilege that was taken away. If you catch your child doing this, inform him or her that the 24-hour period of that privilege loss will now be restarted.

PRACTICE EXERCISE

*One way to practice the house rules is to use Option 1 in Strategy 3 for a few days before using Option 2 or 3. For example, suppose you rated your child as a "1" or "2" on the **How Well Was I Following the House Rules Today?** chart that day for two house rules. You could then warn your child that had you been using automatic time-out (Option 2 in Strategy 3) or removing privileges (Option 3 in Strategy 3), it would have been enforced accordingly. Then you could remind your child that on [specified future date] the automatic time-out or removing privileges for a day will be enforced for house rule violations. This practicing can also serve the purpose of making a gradual transition from having few house rules to enforcing them.*

TROUBLESHOOTING TIP

Parents sometimes ask what they should do if a child earned privileges that day, if using the same-day method, or the day before, if using the next-day method, but then violated a house rule. Should the child continue to have access to the privileges that were previously earned even though a house rule is now being violated? In most cases the answer is "yes." The child earned the privileges, and that "contract" should still be honored if you want to encourage rule following.

Keep in mind that the house rules procedure is a long-term behavior management strategy. It is unrealistic to expect it to work fast or every day. The child will gradually learn to follow house rules as the procedure is applied persistently and consistently over time.

There are exceptions, however, to this general principle. If a child exhibits extreme behavior such as violence, property destruction, or running away on a given day, then all privileges could be suspended immediately for the remainder of that day and the next. Do this sparingly, however, or the incentive to follow house rules to get back privileges will be reduced.

USING SITUATIONAL RULES

You can also use rules for situational challenges inside and outside the house. These rules can be helpful at particular times and/or places where your child's behavior is predictably problematic. **First write down up to four rules for certain situations.** For example:

- **Restaurant rules**—use quiet voice, be polite, use good table manners, stay in your seat.
- **Shopping rules**—use quiet voice, stay by Dad's side, walk and don't run, no candy or toys.
- **Dinner rules**—use quiet voice, use good table manners, turn off cell phone, try everything on your plate.
- **Rules at Grandma's house**—use quiet voice, drink only one can of pop, talk to Grandma politely, use good table manners.
- **Video game rules**—1 hour maximum per day, only after homework is done, avoid non-parent-approved games, allow your sister to join in.
- **Internet rules**—1 hour maximum per day, avoid non-parent-approved sites, do not purchase anything online, avoid specified chat rooms.
- **Rules for going out on weekend nights (for teens)**—follow four W's (see Chapter 11), avoid drinking/drugs, go only to homes where parents are present, no more than four people in the car.

Then review these rules before and after the situation. The review before the situation/event helps remind your child of what is expected and provides some goals for him or her to work on in that specific situation. The review after provides some feedback about how well the child did. You could use a rating format using *1* (Not at all), *2* (A little), *3* (Pretty good), and *4* (Great) to aid in the review. Another option is to tell your child that he or she can earn or lose a specified privilege for following the rules in that situation (similar to Option 3 for making privileges contingent on following house rules, above).

Strategy 4: Managing Your Child's Protests of Time-Out or Removal of Privileges

It is not uncommon for a child to protest (act up) when a parent attempts to use time-out or to remove privileges. This protesting, which can range from sighing and groaning to talking back to throwing chairs, **is an additional target behavior on top of the rule violations, and it warrants its own strategy.** The general idea for handling protests is to ignore them, avoid arguing, and **patiently** follow through with time-out or privilege removal. This does not mean giving in and letting the child have his or her way. It means following through without getting involved in power struggles. It also means **disengaging and deescalating** (e.g., separating, avoiding verbal debates or power struggles, staying calm) if the protesting gets out of hand. **When you are targeting house rules with strategies in this chapter, you will probably need to target child protesting with strategies in Chapter 7 at the same time.**

Achieving Success with Rule Following

The primary goal of this chapter is to get your child to follow rules (parents' behavioral expectations) without always having to be told and without a lot of arguing, talking back, acting up, and so on. This chapter provides ideas and strategies for getting your child to follow designated house rules on a regular basis. To follow through, periodically review the *Parent Checklist for Child Rule Following* at the end of this chapter or set your own goals to attain with the *Parenting Goals* form at the end of Chapter 3.

Keep in mind that sometimes a child's behavior will get worse before it improves when using house rules. Be sure to stay with it. You need to be **persistent** and **consistent** (i.e., PERCON) in applying these skills-building strategies every day until they work. Sometimes this takes weeks or months.

Parent Checklist for Child Rule Following

Name: _____ Date: _____

In the blanks below, indicate a score for **how well** you make use of each parenting behavior at this time.

Not too well	Okay	Very well
1	2	3

Parent's Use of a Positive Approach to Increase Child's Rule Following

A. ____ Building a relationship and bond

B. ____ Avoiding the use of critical or negative comments

C. ____ Catching 'em following the rules by using three positive comments or praise for the child's rule following for every one correction/reprimand for not following them

Parent's Use of Clearly Stated House Rules for Child

D. ____ Discussing house rules so that the child definitely knows them

E. ____ Writing down house rules in clear terms and posting them

Parent's Use of a Firm Approach to Reduce Child's Rule Violations

F. ____ Periodically reviewing the house rules

G. ____ Putting a younger child in automatic time-out for house rules violations

H. ____ Providing access to privileges according to how well the child or teen has followed house rules

Parent's Use of Strategies to Manage Child's Protesting of Discipline for Breaking Rules

I. ____ Ignoring and not getting caught up in the child's talking back, acting up, complaining, and so on, when trying to get the child to follow house rules (see Chapter 7 for more information)

J. ____ Disengaging from power struggles and avoiding yelling, threatening, forcing, and so on, to get the child to follow house rules (see Chapter 7 for more information)

K. ____ Following through with D–H above in a calm manner (see Chapter 7 for more information)

How Well Was I Following the House Rules Today?

1. I think I was following the rules . . .

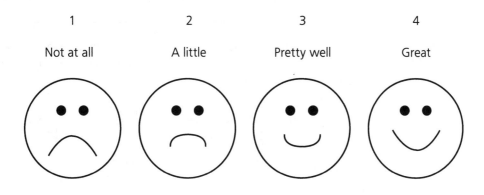

2. You think I was following the rules . . .

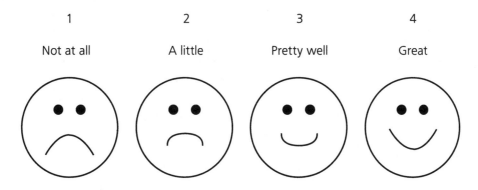

Daily Privileges for Following House Rules

Name: _____

Write down daily time period for which house rules must be followed and when earned privileges can be accessed (e.g., same day or next day): _____

Write down four house rules to be followed each day. Put a Y (Yes) in the box if the rule was followed or an N (No) in the box if the rule was not followed. At the end of the day, tally up the Y's and then provide privileges that were earned that day or the next day.

House rules	Mon.	Tues.	Wed.	Thurs.	Fri.	Sat.	Sun.
1.							
2.							
3.							
4.							
Total Y's (Yes) for the day							

Daily Privileges Earned

4 Y's (Yes) for Level A Privileges = _____ privileges

2–3 Y's (Yes) for Level B Privileges = _____ privileges

0–1 Y (Yes) for Level C Privileges = _____ privileges

6 Doing the Right Thing

Teaching Your Child to Behave Honestly

Honesty involves telling the truth and treating others in a fair and honorable manner. It is highly valued in most families and is indicative of a person's moral character. So naturally parents will become justifiably concerned when their child develops the habit of **lying, sneaking, cheating,** or **stealing.** A certain amount of these behaviors is normal, but over time most children learn that they are wrong and eventually curtail them. If your child has not outgrown these dishonest behaviors, it may be wise to take action. Not only does dishonesty often have immediate negative consequences, but habitual dishonesty erodes trust between the child and family or peers and can cause serious relationship problems both now and in the future.

Children develop a habit of dishonest behavior along a variety of routes. Knowing why your child is behaving in these ways can help you determine how much work you might have to do to reduce his or her dishonesty. Some children exhibit **impulsive dishonesty**; they react with a lie if caught misbehaving, or they sneak or cheat or steal on the spur of the moment without thinking of the consequences. Other children display **peer-pressured dishonesty,** such as when a child is influenced to behave dishonestly by friends or classmates and/or thinks "everyone else is doing it, so why not me?" Perhaps the most serious problem exists when children **value dishonesty,** thinking it's okay or even a good idea to get what they want through dishonest means.

This chapter provides ideas and strategies for teaching a child to be honest. Youth who are more impulsive and/or who are peer pressured may need some of the strategies described, while those who also value dishonesty may require many, if not all, of them.

Choosing a Focus for Honesty

Start by evaluating yourself on the *Parent Checklist for Child Honesty* (at the end of this chapter), which will help you pinpoint where you are now and focus on what needs work. This checklist will also provide an overview of the topics covered in this chapter. You can refer to the same checklist periodically as a reminder and to measure your progress.

Strategy 1: Increasing Your Child's Honesty with a Positive Approach

Your child's honesty can be enhanced if you begin with, and intentionally focus on, a positive approach.

Building a Better Relationship and Avoiding Critical or Negative Comments

It makes sense that having a positive relationship with your child and keeping the everyday communication positive can promote honesty in him or her. Regular bonding activities—almost anything that you and your child can enjoy together, with your child getting your undivided attention—can go a long way toward improving your relationship. Reminding yourself to avoid negative communication (avoiding criticizing the child for the "small stuff," keeping your tone of voice calm even when aggravated, and so forth) will also help, since a pattern of negative comments from you can create distance between the two of you. The investment in building a relationship and fostering everyday communications will pay off in increasing your child's rule-following behavior as well (see Chapter 4 for more details).

Catching 'Em Being Honest

Every child is honest sometimes! Be sure to notice, comment, and praise your child for behaving honestly. For example:

- "I really appreciate it, [child's name], when you tell me the truth."
- "Thank you, [child's name], for staying in the house after school today and not sneaking out to John's house."
- "[Child's name], I really liked it when you played Monopoly fairly and by the rules with your sister."

Strive to offer at least three positive comments and/or praise related to your child's honest behavior for every correction of, or reprimand for, dishonesty!

BUILDING OTHER SOCIAL CONNECTIONS

Building attachments and bonds between your child and other positive people and positive places can promote honesty in him or her. Emphasize involvement in family activities. Try to promote friendships with peers who have a positive-influence and get your child engaged in positive activities at school or in the community or in places of worship (see Chapter 11 for more ideas).

Strategy 2: Reducing Your Child's Dishonesty with a Firm Approach

Parents need a consistent and predictable way of handling incidences of lying, sneaking, cheating, and stealing when they occur. The steps that follow are designed to help you send a message to your child that there are consequences for wrongdoing and to help him or her develop a desire to avoid dishonest behavior in the future. **It is very important that you remain cool and calm while implementing these steps** (see Chapter 18 about ways to stay calm when your child is stressing you out).

Step 1: Noting That the Dishonest Behavior Occurred

The specific incident of lying, sneaking, cheating, or stealing has to be acknowledged publicly. Ideally your child would admit it or you would have concrete evidence that it occurred (e.g., you saw it or there was a witness). Ask your child about the specific incidence of lying, sneaking, cheating, or stealing that you suspect. Sometimes a "5-minute delayed answer" method can be useful, especially for children who lie impulsively or reactively due to immediate fears that they are about to receive a consequence. To do this, tell your child what you suspect (e.g., "I think you stole some money from my purse") and that you will return in 5 minutes to ask him or her about it (e.g., "I'll be back in 5 minutes to ask you if you did this, so think about how you want to answer the question"). Hopefully during the 5-minute break your child will calm down a bit and ponder an honest answer. Then return to your child to ask him or her about the suspected incidence of dishonesty. You can also remind him or her about the consequences of lying (i.e., that the consequence is doubled for lying—see Step 2).

Unfortunately, sometimes a child with a pattern of dishonesty does not tell the truth when caught, and then you have to take additional action. In this instance **it is okay to use your gut reaction as "proof."** If you strongly suspect that lying, sneaking, cheating, or stealing has occurred, it probably has, and it should be treated as if it has. You then tell your child that you think it did occur, and you proceed to Step 2.

 TROUBLESHOOTING TIP
Sometimes a sticky situation emerges where your gut reaction is that your child was dishonest, yet you have no tangible evidence, and your child adamantly denies it. Do not get involved in debates or power struggles trying to prove whether or not the behavior has occurred or respond to how "unfair" you are. Explain to your child that he or she has established an unfortunate pattern of being dishonest in the past and now he or she cannot be trusted fully. Explain further that your child can change this "reputation" by being honest and forthright in the future.

Step 2: Providing a Consequence for Dishonesty

The goal is to **teach a lesson, not to punish**. Establish different levels of consequences depending on whether or not your child eventually owns up to the specific instance of lying, sneaking, cheating, or stealing, including:

Mild Consequence If the Infraction Is Eventually Admitted

Tell your child that he or she will be put in time-out (younger child) or lose a privilege (older child or teen) for lying, sneaking, cheating, or stealing but that the loss of privilege will be less if the child tells the truth (see Chapter 4 for a refresher on time-out and/or removing privileges). For example, the child could be put in time-out or lose a privilege for up to 24 hours, but if he or she continues to deny it, the consequence would be longer. Privileges that could be removed include access to video games, computer, television, cell phone, sports equipment (e.g., bicycle, basketball, hockey skates), iPod, going out with friends, or the car for an older teen.

Moderate Consequence If the Infraction Continues to Be Denied

Tell your child that he or she will be put in time-out or lose the privilege for double the time of above. This means that the time-out will be twice as long or the removal of privileges will be for 48 hours because the child did not "own up to it."

> ## AVOID SEVERE CONSEQUENCES
>
> There is some research to suggest that a child who habitually engages in forms of dishonest behavior is not affected by severe consequences or punishments. Severe consequences can backfire in that the child may focus only on that (e.g., "she is so mean") and rationalize continuing the behavior in the future (e.g., "I have to sneak because he is so unfair"). Instead of severe consequences try to follow through with mild or moderate consequences for each act of dishonesty on a consistent basis until you see progress.

Step 3: Arranging an Apology and Restitution

Your child should be expected to apologize to the "victim" of this instance of lying, sneaking, cheating, or stealing and make it up to that person. After apologizing, the child should perform extra chores, do extra favors, and/or pay a "fine." If the infraction involved stealing, the child should also be required to return or replace the stolen item.

Step 4: Helping the Child Understand How Dishonesty Impacts Others

This can be accomplished by clearly communicating disappointment in your child and by requiring a discussion (or written essay from older child or teen) on how the child's behavior impacted others. Ask the child to state how others might have thought and felt and whether he or she wants to be trusted by others. Sometimes it can help to utilize role reversal by asking what it would feel like if the same thing happened to the child.

It may be necessary to repeat the four steps over and over with your child before they have an impact. Unfortunately, it sometimes takes a while to learn from one's mistakes.

 PRACTICE EXERCISES
It is very helpful to Practice steps 1–4 to instill honesty in your child. It may help to recall a past episode of lying, sneaking, cheating, or stealing and role-

play it using the steps with your practitioner or with a parenting partner (if applicable). The adults would take turns acting as the "child" and the "parent." Then, if your child is cooperative, you two could do some role playing. You and your child can act out the steps to practice and to help your child understand what will be occurring at home in the future. These role plays with the child can be tricky, so it may be best to do them with a practitioner's assistance.

Strategy 3: Promoting the Development of Your Child's Honesty

The development of honesty involves gradually learning what is right and wrong and being concerned with how one's behavior affects others. Children first learn to follow "external rules" imposed by others and then over time gradually develop their own set of "internal rules" to guide their behavior. Several skills-building parenting strategies can be applied to promote the development of honesty in your child.

Promoting Rule Following

For the child who is struggling "internally" with doing the right thing, it can be helpful to "externally" make him or her follow rules to stay out of trouble (especially with sneaky behavior). Make sure that your house rules are well known to the child and that you follow through with consequences when he or she violates them (see Chapter 5 for more details).

Increasing Parental Monitoring

A child who is engaging in dishonest behavior may need to be monitored to keep him or her out of trouble (especially with sneaky behavior). To do this, make sure you always know the "four W's"—**what** your child is doing, **whom** your child is with, **where** your child is going, and **when** your child will be home each time he or she goes out (see Chapter 11 for more details). Keeping tabs on your child in this way affords him or her fewer opportunities for dishonest behavior.

PEER PRESSURE COPING SKILLS

The influence of peers can be powerful. As indicated earlier, some children succumb to peer pressure and behave dishonestly. Promoting rule following and increasing parental monitoring can reduce negative peer influence, but they may not be enough. Some children benefit from learning coping skills for dealing with peer pressure, which involves ways to avoid peer pressure situations or to be assertive when pressured by peers. See Chapter 11 for more details about teaching a child peer pressure coping skills.

Redirecting to Honest Ways of Getting Things

By lying, sneaking, cheating, or stealing, your child may be trying to get what he or she wants "through the back door." It can be helpful to redirect the child who seems to value or prefer dishonest ways of getting things to go "through the front door" instead. This means coming up with ways that your child can earn what he or she wants in positive and accepted ways. This can be accomplished by setting up an allowance, directing the teen to get a job, giving increasing privileges as he or she proves trustworthy, etc. Be clear in telling your child what he or she needs to do to earn your trust and regain privileges.

PROMOTING THE VALUE OF HONESTY AND DOING RIGHT BY OTHERS

Make honesty an important family value. To do this, parents need to be role models for honesty, talk about the importance of honesty, acknowledge how difficult it is to be honest at times, and discuss situations that come up in terms of "doing the right thing." Prompt your child to discuss situations where he or she may have resisted temptation to be dishonest and instead behaved honestly (e.g., after you asked, your son reported seeing a lady walk away, leaving a purse behind, and informed her of it). This latter suggestion is also in keeping with Catching 'Em Being Honest and deserves praise.

Strategy 4: Managing Your Child's Protests with Time-Out or Removal of Privileges

It is not uncommon for a child to protest (act up) when a parent attempts to use time-out or to remove privileges. This protesting, which can range from sighing and groaning to talking back to throwing chairs, **is an additional target behavior on top of the dishonesty, and it warrants its own strategy.** The general idea for handling protests is to ignore them, avoid arguing, and **patiently** follow through with time-out or privilege removal. This does not mean giving in and letting the child have his or her way. It means following through without getting involved in power struggles. It also means **disengaging and deescalating** (e.g., separating, avoiding verbal debates or power struggles, staying calm) if the protesting gets out of hand. **When you are targeting dishonesty with strategies in this chapter, you will probably need to target your child's protesting with the strategies in Chapter 7 at the same time.**

Achieving Success with Honesty

Honesty involves telling the truth and treating others in a fair and honorable manner without arguing, talking back, acting up, and so on. This chapter provides ideas and strategies to help your child to be more truthful and honest. To follow through, it is highly recommended that you periodically review the *Parent Checklist for Child Honesty* at the end of this chapter or set your own goals to attain with the *Parenting Goals* form at the end of Chapter 3.

Be prepared, because sometimes children struggling with dishonesty are defensive. Such a child may blame you and have a hard time accepting responsibility. You will "teach" the child by following through with the actions described in this chapter, and hopefully over time your child will internalize honest behavioral standards. This will be achieved only if you stay with it. You need to be **persistent** and **consistent** (i.e., PERCON) in applying these skills-building strategies every day until they work. Sometimes this takes weeks or months.

Parent Checklist for Child Honesty

Name: _____ Date: _____

In the blanks below, indicate a score for **how well** you make use of that parenting behavior at this time.

Not too well	Okay	Very well
1	2	3

Parent's Use of a Positive Approach to Increase Child's Honesty

A. ____ Building a relationship and bond

B. ____ Avoiding the use of critical or negative comments

C. ____ Catching 'em being honest by using three positive comments or praise related to the child's honest behavior for every one correction/reprimand for dishonest behavior

Parent's Use of a Firm Approach When Child's Dishonesty Occurs

D. ____ Publicly acknowledging the specific incidence of dishonesty either by the child's admitting it or by your saying it occurred based on a "gut reaction"

E. ____ Providing a mild consequence (e.g., remove privileges for 24 hours) if dishonesty is admitted or a moderate consequence (e.g., remove privileges for 48 hours) if dishonesty is denied

F. ____ Making sure that the child apologizes and makes restitution to the "victim" of dishonesty

G. ____ Communicating disappointment and reviewing how the dishonest behavior impacted others

Parent's Use of Strategies to Promote Development of Child's Honesty

H. ____ Enforcing clearly defined house rules

I. ____ Keeping close tabs on the child through monitoring, including when out of house

J. ____ Promoting the child's earning what is wanted instead of getting it dishonestly

Parent's Use of Strategies to Manage Child's Protesting of Discipline for Dishonesty

K. ____ Ignoring and not getting caught up in the child's talking back, acting up, complaining, and so on, when trying to teach the child to behave honestly (see Chapter 7 for more information)

L. ____ Disengaging from power struggles and avoiding yelling, threatening, forcing, and so on to teach the child to behave honestly (see Chapter 7 for more information)

M. ____ Following through with D–J above in a calm manner (see Chapter 7 for more information)

7

Staying Cool under Fire

Managing Your Child's Protesting of Discipline
and Preventing Angry Outbursts

Among the most difficult child behaviors to deal with is an episode of angry and confrontational behavior that comes up in the spur of the moment. This volatility is often a protest triggered by a parent's attempt to discipline the child for misbehavior and/or some disagreement where the child thinks he or she is being treated unfairly. Parents often feel ill-equipped to handle this hostility because it happens so fast and is so intense. It is stressful for both child and parent. When the dust settles, it is common for a child and parent to feel bad about each other and sometimes regret what was said and done. Teaching children ways to calm themselves internally is the subject of Chapter 14. This chapter is about managing a child's protests and preventing angry outbursts externally—through your own parenting efforts.

Note: *This chapter focuses on a very tough problem. Although the methods described will undoubtedly help if they are applied faithfully, it may not be enough. Additional child-focused skills such as those in the emotional development section (Chapters 12–14), parent-focused skills like those designed to enhance your well-being (Chapters 17–18), or family-focused skills that can promote your family's well-being (Chapters 19–20) may also be helpful. Be sure to work with your practitioner on this challenging problem, both to facilitate skills development and to consider other mental health interventions, as needed.*

Choosing a Focus for Protesting and Angry Outbursts

Start by using the *Parent Checklist for Child Protests and Angry Outbursts* (at the end of this chapter) to pinpoint where you are now and focus on what needs work. This checklist will also provide an overview of the topics covered in this chapter.

You can refer to the checklist, periodically as needed, for reminders and to measure your progress.

Strategy 1: Increasing Calmness in Your Child with a Positive Approach

Your child's calmness can be enhanced if you begin with, and intentionally focus on, a positive approach.

Building a Better Relationship and Avoiding Critical or Negative Comments

Having a good relationship with your child and routinely making constructive comments to him or her can go a long way toward preventing angry outbursts. When children know they can trust their parents' love and goodwill, they don't view their parents as adversaries every time the parents exercise their authority. Unfortunately, a history of protests and anger from your child could very well have weakened the bond of trust between the two of you and resulted in a negative pattern of everyday communication. It is good idea to make a concerted effort to reestablish a rapport with your child and to make fewer negative and more constructive comments to your child (see Chapter 4 for more details).

Catching 'Em Staying Calm

Even children who frequently get upset stay calm sometimes! You may be in the habit of staying quiet yourself at those times, for fear of upsetting the applecart if you remark on your child's behavior at all. But noticing, commenting, and praising your child for staying calm during a moment that typically elicits anger calls for a positive reaction from you. For example:

- "Thank you, [child's name], for staying calm when I told you to come in from outside."

- "[Child's name], I really liked it when you kept your cool after I took away your TV privileges for not coming in on time."

- "I really appreciated it, [child's name], when you stayed calm as we reviewed the house rules."

Strive to offer at least three positive comments and/or praise related to your child's staying calm for every correction or reprimand for protests or outbursts!

Strategy 2: Managing Protesting When Disciplining Your Child

Chapters 4, 5, and 6 described procedures for reducing your child's noncompliant, rule-violating, and/or dishonest behaviors, respectively. Time-out and/or removal of privileges were recommended for handling such misbehavior, but angry resistance of these consequences can occur for some children. **This protesting is an additional target behavior on top of the original misbehavior, and it warrants its own strategy.**

When it comes to protesting, you have three choices: (1) **give in** and let your child have his or her way, (2) use a **power tactic** (yelling, physically forcing, etc.) to make your child go to time-out or relinquish a privilege, or (3) take a **patient approach** of deferring the time-out or privilege removal until your child is calm (described below). Choice 1 is ill-advised because giving in reinforces the protesting behavior. Choice 2 is not good because it can escalate power struggles, create bad feelings between you and your child, and inadvertently "teach" the child to overreact when disciplined. Choice 3 is arguably best because you are eventually following through in a calm manner. In addition, you are modeling how to stay calm when using the patient approach.

The general idea for handling protests is to ignore them and *patiently* **follow through with time-out or privilege removal while avoiding power struggles.** This approach teaches your child that you mean business because you eventually follow through with discipline, and you are modeling staying calm. This matter of staying calm is, of course, much easier said than done, so careful application of the steps below is essential. It is also important to have realistic expectations. The ideas here will not suddenly change a child's volatile behavior. But using these ideas over time will very gradually reduce the number, length, and intensity of the outbursts in most children.

Managing Mild Protesting with Ignoring

Some children protest *mildly*—grunting and groaning, huffing and puffing, talking under their breath, and the like. If your child goes to time-out or gives up the privilege you designated, but complains while doing so, **the best response is to** *ignore* **this by looking away and avoiding discussion of this behavior.**

Managing Moderate Protesting with Ignoring *and* Patient Standoff

Some children protest *moderately*—banging things, yelling very loudly, getting out of the time-out chair, and/or refusing to comply with privilege removal. **At this point it's best to postpone the time-out or privilege removal until your child calms down.** This entails ignoring protesting behaviors and going into the **patient standoff** mode. The goal of the patient standoff is to remain calm, avoid power struggles, and eventually "win," manifested by your child's doing what you warned would be the consequence. Avoid power tactics to get your child to comply, such as yelling, threatening, or getting physical. The patient standoff also involves **disengaging** and **deescalating** if the protesting gets out of hand (see Strategy 3).

Patient Standoff When Using Time-Out

Warn your child that you can't start the timer, or you'll have to reset it, if the protesting continues. If your child refuses to sit in time-out, tell the child that a privilege like TV, video games, or a bicycle will be removed until the child does the time-out (e.g., "No TV until you do your time-out"). If your child will not relinquish these privileges (e.g., won't stop watching TV), then you could "go on strike" (see below). When your child is calm, ask if he or she is ready to begin time-out. If "yes," then follow through; if "no," continue the patient standoff. **Be forewarned: It can take a long time to get even a moderately protesting child to complete a time-out!**

Patient Standoff When Using Privilege Removal

Warn your child that he or she cannot have the privilege, or you cannot start the 24-hour privilege restriction (depending on which option you used in the warning), until he or she gives up that privilege (e.g., hands over the phone, stops watching TV, gets off of the computer). Tell the child that the privilege will be removed for 24 hours beginning when the privilege is surrendered. If your child will not relinquish the privileges (e.g., won't stop watching TV), then you could "go on strike" (see below). When your child is calm, ask if he or she is ready to begin the privilege removal. If "yes," follow through; if "no," continue the patient standoff.

 TROUBLESHOOTING TIP
It can help to "go on strike" when using the patient standoff but your child will not give up a privilege (e.g., won't turn off TV). Instead of arguing or forc-

ing your child to give up a privilege you can temporarily stop all of the nice things you do for your child, including chauffeuring, ironing clothes, cooking special foods, and helping the child in various ways. These "extras" are in fact privileges you give your child that can be removed by telling him or her "I am going on strike until you [relinquish privilege]" (e.g., turn off TV). Then stop doing extra nice things until the child cooperates. Understand, however, that going on strike should never involve abdicating your parental responsibility to keep your child fed, clothed, sheltered, and healthy. So-called nice things that you do for your child are those optional favors that the child can live, safely and healthily, without.

One caution is to use the "on strike" method in moderation. If your child digs in his or her heels for an extended period of time and will still not give up the privilege, then it is wise to suspend the strike and try other methods in consultation with your practitioner.

Managing Severe Protesting with Ignoring *and* Patient Standoff *and* Safety Precautions

Some children protest **severely**—threatening others, throwing things, hitting, etc. The preceding methods still apply, but you also need to **take precautions to ensure that everyone is safe.** Ideally you will deescalate and disengage (see Strategy 3) and simultaneously monitor your child. This is accomplished best by calmly walking away from your child while keeping an eye on him or her from a safe distance to prevent potential harm to self, others, or property.

Your child may be so upset, however, that he or she follows you or ramps up the protests even more to draw you in. If this occurs, you could try sending your child to his or her room to "cool down" (not as punishment), telling the child that the time-out or privilege removal will still be imposed once calm. If severe protesting starts again, then it is back to the room to cool down. Keep doing this until a calm time-out is eventually served or the privilege removal is accepted calmly. Strive to give your child positive attention for calming down and then complying with your discipline, once he or she does so.

Very rarely the preceding measures fail and the safety of a child or others becomes a concern. **If needed, isolate and remove others from the severely protesting child and get help.** Sometimes, as a last resort, it is necessary to restrain a younger child or call the police for an older child. You have to supervise your child and stay calm at all times. If your child has a habit of placing self or others at personal risk because of severe protesting, it is highly recommended that you consult with your practitioner about other mental health interventions that may be needed.

AVOID ADDING ON MORE CONSEQUENCES

It's tempting to give your child more consequences during the protest phase because he or she is talking back and you are angry (e.g., "That talking back just earned you another day without your computer!"). This tactic, unfortunately, can make matters worse. It usually escalates power struggles and makes it hard to follow through. Instead, try handling protests as described in this section. Remember that each time you effectively manage the protests, you'll see less and less of them over time.

It's also tempting to give your child more consequences for continued noncompliance (e.g., "Okay, now you have 24 more hours since you are now refusing to turn off the computer!"). But this also is ineffective. It can create a sticky situation of more and more arguing, and again it will be hard to follow through. Instead, each time your child is noncompliant, simply put the child back in time-out or inform the child that the 24 hours of privilege removal begins anew.

TROUBLESHOOTING TIP

*At this stage parents sometimes lose their cool and occasionally resort to "power tactics" (e.g., yelling, threatening, nagging, physically forcing) to deal with protests. This is an understandable response given how upsetting and frustrating a protesting child can be, but such power tactics often do more harm than good. They can lead to escalation in that moment and bad feelings between the child and parent over time. Instead, calmly keep following the steps to deal with protesting outlined in this chapter. **Remember that patience wins over power in the long run, even though this may involve continuing the process over many weeks or months before you see results.***

Strategy 3: Disengaging and Deescalating When Your Child Is Agitated

It is very important to **disengage** and **deescalate** when dealing with an agitated (upset, angry, irritated, etc.) child. This does not mean that you should walk away and let the child "win." It means that everyone has to calm down, after which you go back to dealing with the child's misbehavior.

There are several benefits to this disengaging and deescalating process. First, any disciplining you are doing will go more smoothly and quickly if you stay cool and focused. Second, many children who get upset easily have emotion regulation challenges, and if you can stay calm, your child will learn to calm down more rapidly. You'll notice that it takes your child less and less time to calm down each time you do this. **Disengaging and deescalating are most effectively done verbally, physically, and emotionally.**

Verbally Disengaging and Deescalating

The key here is to cut down on what you say and change the way you talk to your child when the child is agitated.

- Avoid debates, explanations, and/or justifying why you are doing what you are doing. Try not to get caught up in unproductive back-and-forth retorts, often escalating discussions about how "unfair" you are.

- It is okay to use *"I understand" statements* to acknowledge your child's feelings (e.g., "I see that you are frustrated," "I heard you say that I am unfair," "I know how important this is to you").

- It is also okay to use the *"broken record technique"* of restating your expectations (e.g., "I'll talk to you after you do your time-out," "As soon as you calm down and do the dishes, you can watch TV," "After you calm down and clean up the mess you made, we can talk about it").

Physically Disengaging and Deescalating

Physically disengaging and deescalating is best done by walking away. If your child follows you, at least try to say less—the less you say, the better—and minimize eye contact.

Emotionally Disengaging and Deescalating

This boils down to staying calm! Try these suggestions to help you:

- Think coping thoughts, such as, "I'm going to stay calm," "I won't let him or her get to me," "I can do it," "Take some deep breaths," etc.

- Relax your body by taking deep breaths, counting to 10, etc.

- **Imagine yourself as a robot!** Like a robot, get the child to complete time-out or give up a privilege while staying cool.

Keeping your cool is the key to disengaging and deescalating. See Chapter 18 for more ideas for staying calm during stressful parent–child interactions.

 PRACTICE EXERCISE
This business of staying calm while enforcing discipline is hard to do, so it requires practice. One way to practice is to do role plays simulating typical scenarios that bring on your child's protesting and then react by managing mild, moderate, or severe protesting and by using the disengaging and deescalating strategies. You could role-play using the procedures with your practitioner or with a parenting partner (if applicable). If your child is cooperative, do some more role playing with him or her. This will also be good preparation for your child, and then he or she will not be surprised when you actually use the strategies. It is highly recommended that you undertake such role plays under the guidance of your practitioner, because they can be difficult to do correctly.

Strategy 4: Emphasizing the Prevention of Angry Outbursts

This may be the most effective strategy of all because you prevent the outbursts in the first place.
A child goes through four stages in the angry outburst process. The best way to deal with an angry outburst is to prevent it from escalating in the early stages. This can be accomplished by emphasizing the **proactive** strategies at Stages 1 and 2. If an outburst occurs despite these efforts, the **reactive** strategies will be necessary at Stages 3 and 4.

Stage 1: Maintaining a State of Calm

- *Child functioning.* This is everyday routine behavior where your child is emotionally calm and engaging in productive behavior and interactions with others.

- *Proactive parent response.* To maintain this calm state in your child, it is a good idea to have predictable household routines and clearly stated rules and expectations and to pay attention to positive behaviors in your child (see Chapters 5 and

19 for detailed suggestions). This kind of routine and structure reduces problem behaviors, which means that you have to discipline your child less often and, in turn, your child has fewer opportunities to protest.

Stage 2: Redirecting an Increasingly Agitated Child

• *Child functioning.* Your child reacts to a stressful situation and/or "trigger" (your discipline, disagreements, pressures, mistakes, etc.) with agitation. He or she may show increased emotional arousal (e.g., irritated, upset, worried, frustrated) and/or unfocused behavior (e.g., staring, poor eye contact, just standing there). There may be escalating behaviors that engage others in conflict (e.g., arguing, provoking comments, whining, verbal abuse).

• *Proactive parent response.* Use calming strategies such as recognizing your child's feelings (e.g., "I see that you look upset") and/or guiding your child to use stress management (see Chapter 14) and/or to participate in a family cool-down, where everyone separates briefly to calm down (see Chapter 20). **However, prompting a child to use stress management or participate in a family cool-down will not work unless the child has been trained in those skills.** It can backfire if you prompt the child to use a skill he or she doesn't really have. If your son or daughter knows how to use those skills, however, there is a better chance that he or she will be able to calm down and move out of this agitation phase.

As your child gets increasingly agitated you should also allow yourself the space and time to calm down, avoid escalating verbal statements and power struggles, and try to stay detached. Getting upset can make your child more volatile. The basic idea is to stay firm in your expectations while also patiently trying to create a calm atmosphere.

Stage 3: Dealing with the Angry Outburst

• *Child functioning.* The child is very upset and aggressive. This could include threats to the child's own safety and/or the safety of others, destruction of property, and/or physical assault.

• *Reactive parent response.* At this point you are doing crisis management, which entails simultaneously **disengaging and deescalating while maintaining safety.** This is challenging because to maintain safety, you may have to interact with your child. See the earlier sections on disengaging/deescalating and safety.

Stage 4: Recovery from the Angry Outburst

• *Child functioning.* The outburst is declining and the child is returning to calm.

• *Reactive parent response.* Once calm, it is your child's responsibility to clean up and make restitution if applicable (e.g., pay for damages, do extra chores, apologize). It may also be a good idea to process what happened, as long as your child stays calm when doing so. This may be a good time to discuss the underlying feelings of sadness, anxiety, or stress that may be at the root of the outburst. If your child is agreeable, it may also help to discuss stress management techniques (see Chapter 14).

In summary, a child goes through four predictable stages on the way to an angry outburst. The main point is for parents to recognize the stages and respond accordingly. **I strongly advise that you try to prevent the outbursts in the first place by emphasizing the proactive strategies at Stages 1 and 2.**

STOPPING THE NAGGING THAT CAN TRIGGER CONFLICT

Here is an additional tip that can be used to avoid or minimize parent–child conflict. Every now and then a child will ask for something. If you are vague in responding to the request, often to avoid a conflict, the child may nag you to give in. These kinds of interactions, where the parent is unclear and the child keeps nagging, can stimulate conflict.

One way to avoid endless nagging and "negotiations" from your child is by being firm and clear in responding to requests. The **"Traffic Signal Answer Technique"** can be used to nip the nagging in the bud. In response to a request, you can say:

- **"Green:** Yes, it's a go."
- **"Yellow:** Let's discuss it further."
- **"Red:** Absolutely not, and I will not change my mind, and I will not discuss it further."

Adding the traffic signal category to the answer makes your response very clear. It may not be received very positively when you begin using it, but over time your child will come to clearly understand your answers to requests, and this clarity and firmness will reduce conflict.

Achieving Success with Protesting and Angry Outbursts

Protests and outbursts occur when a child is highly agitated in response to a parent's directives and/or discipline. This chapter provides ideas and strategies for calming down parent–child interactions when your child balks at your discipline or gets upset. To follow through, I highly recommend that you periodically review the *Parent Checklist for Child Protests and Angry Outbursts* at the end of this chapter or set your own goals to attain with the *Parenting Goals* form at the end of Chapter 3.

Keep in mind that the highly volatile child is likely struggling with emotional regulation, and therefore might take a fair amount of time to calm him or her down. Although protesting and angry outbursts may not go away as fast as you'd like, you should see that the episodes are shorter and shorter in duration over time. You need to be **persistent** and **consistent** (i.e., PERCON) in applying these skills-building strategies every day until it works, and sometimes it takes weeks or months.

Parent Checklist for Child Protests and Angry Outbursts

Name: _____ Date: _____

In the blanks below, indicate a score for **how well** you make use of that parenting behavior at this time.

Not too well	Okay	Very well
1	2	3

Parent's Use of a Positive Approach to Increase Child's Calmness

A. _____ Building a relationship and bond

B. _____ Avoiding the use of critical or negative comments

C. _____ Catching 'em staying calm by using three positive comments or praise related to staying calm for every one correction or reprimand for getting angry or having an outburst

Parent's Use of a Patient Approach to Manage Child's Protesting

D. _____ Managing *mild* child protesting (grunting, complaining, etc.) by ignoring it

E. _____ Managing *moderate* child protesting (refusing to be disciplined, stomping off, slamming the door, etc.) with ignoring, remaining calm, avoiding power struggles, and patiently getting the child to eventually do what he or she was told (i.e., a "patient standoff")

F. _____ Managing *severe* protesting with ignoring, patiently prevailing, and taking safety precautions as needed (isolating and removing others; calling police as last resort)

Parent's Use of Disengaging and Deescalating Techniques with an Agitated Child

G. _____ Reducing unproductive discussions when the child is agitated; making occasional *"I understand" statements* ("I see that you are upset") and using the *"broken record technique"* (repeating "As soon as you calm down, we can discuss it" and so on)

H. _____ Minimizing eye contact and trying to walk away

I. _____ Staying calm!

Parent's Use of Prevention to Avoid or Reduce Child's Angry Outbursts

J. _____ Maintaining a state of calm in the child by using predictable household routines, clearly stated rules, and attending to positive behaviors in the child

K. _____ Redirecting an increasingly agitated child by guiding in the use of stress management and/or family cool-down at first signs of child agitation

L. _____ Dealing with the child's angry outburst by disengaging/deescalating while maintaining safety

M. _____ Helping the child recover by prompting him or her to clean up, possibly make restitution, and process what happened if the child is cooperative

Enhancing Your Child's Social Development

8

Making Friends

Teaching Your Child Social Behavior Skills

Many children have difficulty getting along with others. They may display too many negative social behaviors—name calling, interrupting, or being withdrawn, for example—and too few positive social behaviors, such as making eye contact, expressing feelings, and being assertive. This chapter will give you suggestions for teaching and coaching your child in positive social behavior skills.

Choosing a Focus for Social Behaviors

Start by using the *Parent Checklist for Child Social Behaviors* (at the end of this chapter) to pinpoint where you are now and focus on what needs work. This checklist will also provide an overview of the topics covered in this chapter. You can refer to the checklist periodically for reminders and to measure your progress.

Strategy 1: Teaching Your Child Social Behavior Skills

Many children learn social behavior skills on their own, by watching others and through the trial-and-error process of everyday social interactions. Some children, however, need explicit training in these important skills. This section provides step-by-step instructions to enable you to teach your child social behavior skills.

Step 1: Identifying Social Behaviors to Work On

The first task is to figure out which negative social behaviors your child displays too often and which positive social behaviors the child needs help to develop. Think about whether your child shows any of the following negative social behaviors:

- Physical aggression
- Playing unfairly
- Arguing
- Interrupting
- Name calling
- Bossing others
- Whining, complaining, and so forth
- Taking others' possessions
- Dominating the activity
- Making poor eye contact
- Being a poor sport
- Being too loud
- Showing off

- Teasing
- Butting in
- Bugging others
- Getting into others' space
- Withdrawing and isolating self
- Letting others be too bossy
- Listening poorly
- Hoarding food, toys, and so forth
- Keeping feelings inside
- Talking too much
- Disobeying rules of play
- Playing too roughly
- Succumbing to peer pressure

Now it is a good idea to think about alternative positive social behaviors your child could learn to replace the negative social behaviors. The ***Identifying Social Behaviors to Work On*** form (at the end of this chapter) can serve as a starting point. These lists are not exhaustive, and you may be able to think of other social behavior skills that would be useful to target. As you can see, there are two lists of positive social behaviors, one basic and one advanced. These lists will be useful for children and teens at different stages of development. The main point is to select specific social behavior(s) so that you and your child can work on them. It is often useful to get the child's input about the items on the ***Identifying Social Behaviors to Work On*** form too. After careful consideration, choose one or two specific social behaviors to work on with your child.

TROUBLESHOOTING TIP
Knowing where to start can be challenging. If you have the opportunity, spend some time observing your child's interactions with siblings and other peers. Make a note of any interactional problems that may emerge or "social interfering" behaviors that your child might display (e.g., bossy, pushy, too loud, withdrawing, interrupting). Then think of the opposite or replacement behaviors that may be incompatible with the interfering behavior and work with your child on those. For example, you may observe that your child is too loud and interrupts others, in which case you might work on using a quieter inside voice and listening to others.

Step 2: Teaching Social Behaviors to Your Child

Your child needs to learn the specific social behavior you chose. This is accomplished by describing and physically practicing the behavior.

- Explain each social behavior that was chosen (remember, only one or two!).

- Demonstrate what the social behavior looks like.

- Role-play/practice together by taking turns and "acting out" the social behavior(s).

Keep teaching your child the chosen skill until he or she has mastered it in this training context before coaching the child to use it in real life.

 PRACTICE EXERCISE
If your child is working on starting conversations, explain what starting conversations entails, show what starting conversations looks like (you demonstrate it), and then have your child practice starting conversations (the child demonstrates it). You might take turns starting different conversations with each other. Keep this up until your child completely understands and can physically perform the social behavior before moving to the next step.

Step 3: Coaching Social Behaviors in Your Child

You can coach your child to practice the new social behavior skills in everyday interactions with friends, siblings, and/or parents. Social interactions with those people can provide good opportunities to practice social behavior skills.

You can also review and dialogue with your child to create more awareness including:

- Practice the social behavior with your child through role playing.

- Remind your child to use the new social behavior from time to time (ideally, several times a day).

- Discuss daily social interaction events and how the targeted social skill(s) could be useful.

- Be sure to notice, comment, and praise your child for using the social behaviors.

Keep coaching your child on the chosen skill until he or she has mastered it in the real world.

Illustration with Younger Child

If you know that our child will be going to a cousin's birthday party, for example, you might plan ways for him or her to work on sharing during the party. When at the birthday party, you would remind your child to share. Later, your child might receive a reward for doing a good job.

Illustration with Older Child or Teen

If you know that your older child or teen will be going to a family holiday event, for example, you might plan ways for him or her to engage in conversations. Or, if you know that your older child or teen has problems getting along with a sibling each day after school, you might plan ways for him or her to ignore or be assertive

BE A ROLE MODEL OF POSITIVE SOCIAL BEHAVIORS

One of the best ways to teach is to be a good role model of what you are teaching. You too could declare several social behaviors that you will work on and share that with your child (e.g., "I'll work on talking in a brief manner and listening to others"). Then make a point of using those social skills in front of your child and even telling him or her when you are doing it.

(without being aggressive). Later, your older child or teen might receive a reward for doing a good job.

Strategy 2: Creating Social Opportunities for Your Child

A child cannot work on social behavior skills without the opportunity to interact with peers. **Sometimes a child is neglected (ignored) or rejected (rebuffed) by peers. In those cases you may need to assist the child by manufacturing opportunities to be with other children.** With younger children arranging "play dates" is one choice. With older children and teens it may mean orchestrating a sleepover, inviting others over for dinner, weekend camping trips, etc. It is best to start with dyads or small groups and perhaps have a certain amount of adult involvement or supervision. **You could plan how the child will work on social behavior goals prior to the activity and process how well it went afterward.**

Achieving Success with Social Behaviors

To make friends your child must have positive social behaviors in his or her repertoire, such as the ability to share, take turns, be assertive, and negotiate. This chapter provides ideas and strategies with which you can teach and guide your child to develop social behavior skills. To follow through, periodically review the *Parent Checklist for Child Social Behaviors* form at the end of this chapter or set your own goals to attain with the *Parenting Goals* form at the end of Chapter 3. It is also a good idea to encourage your child to set specific social behavior goals ("I will try to share more," "I will work on conversation skills," etc.) and monitor progress on the *Personal Goals (Basic* or *Advanced)* form at the end of Chapter 3. Consider providing rewards to your child for trying the new social behavior skills (see Chapter 3 for more ideas on motivating your child).

The basic social skills usually take several weeks of effort to teach and guide, and the more advanced skills take even longer before they become second nature. You need to be **persistent** and **consistent** (i.e., PERCON) in applying these skills-building strategies every day until they work. Sometimes this takes weeks or months.

Parent Checklist for Child Social Behaviors

Name: _____ **Date:** _____

In the blanks below, indicate a score for **how well** you make use of that parenting behavior at this time.

	Not too well	**Okay**	**Very well**
	1	2	3

Parent's Efforts in Teaching Child Social Behavior Skills

A. ____ Identifying specific social behavior(s) to work on that match the child's age, such as sharing or taking turns or assertiveness or negotiating

B. ____ Teaching specific social behaviors by explaining, demonstrating, and role-playing/practicing of specified social behavior(s) with the child

C. ____ Coaching specific social behavior(s) by periodically reviewing to create more awareness and/or using a chart to promote use of social behavior skill(s)

Parent's Efforts in Creating Social Opportunities for Child

D. ____ Arranging and orchestrating social activities to give the child social opportunities

E. ____ Planning social behavior goals prior to the activity and processing how well it went afterward

Identifying Social Behaviors to Work On

Name: _____ **Date:** _____

Below are lists of basic and advanced positive social behaviors. Circle one or two social behaviors that your child can work on at this time. Put a square around any social behaviors that could be worked on later.

Examples of Basic Social Behaviors

- Taking turns
- Sharing
- Expressing feelings
- Cooperating
- Making eye contact
- Conversing with others
- Listening to others
- Complimenting others
- Accepting compliments
- Following rules of play
- Apologizing to others
- Asking questions
- Using a quieter "inside voice"

- Telling others about self
- Playing fairly
- Inquiring about others' interests
- Talking in a brief manner
- Asking for what one wants/needs
- Helping others
- Inviting others to do something
- Greeting others
- Introducing oneself
- Entering a group
- Getting someone's attention
- Being a good winner/loser
- Other basic social behaviors

Examples of Advanced Social Behaviors

- Respectfully disagreeing with someone
- Compromising with someone
- Ignoring when appropriate
- Being assertive or sticking up for oneself when appropriate
- Displaying social confidence
- Resisting peer pressure
- Negotiating

- Resolving conflicts
- Being aware of how one's behavior affects others
- Being aware of behaviors that irritate others
- Staying calm with others
- Stopping, thinking, and planning to resolve a conflict or disagreement
- Other advanced social behaviors

Write down other social behaviors not listed that might be good to work on:

_____

_____

_____

_____

9

Keeping Friends

Teaching Your Child Social
Problem-Solving Skills

There will always be disagreements and things to work out between your child and others as they interact. Being able to solve social problems can be especially useful for a child who has a track record of not getting along with peers or family members. This chapter offers suggestions for teaching your child to recognize when a social problem exists and to use a step-by-step process to solve the problem.

Choosing a Focus for Social Problem Solving

Start by using the *Parent Checklist for Child Social Problem Solving* (at the end of this chapter) to pinpoint where you are now and focus on what needs work. This checklist will also provide an overview of the topics covered in this chapter. You can refer to the checklist periodically for reminders and to measure your progress.

Strategy 1: Teaching Your Child Social Problem-Solving Skills

Because social problem solving is a complex skill to learn, clear training of these important skills is essential. This section provides step-by-step instructions to enable you to teach your child social problem-solving skills; an experienced practitioner can help you if you get stuck.

Step 1: Discussing and Practicing Social Problem-Solving Skills

Below are two different sequences of the social problem-solving steps, one basic and one advanced. These lists will be useful for children and teens at different stages of development.

Basic Social Problem Solving for a Younger Child

Review the **Basic Social Problem Solving** chart at the end of this chapter. Discuss an example to show how to use each social problem-solving step as shown in the chart. Let's say the example is **"Suppose I am watching a TV show and Michelle turns the channel."**

1. **"Stop! What is the social problem?"**—"I was watching TV, and my sister just turned the channel."

2. **"What are some plans?"**—"I could hit her, I could ask her to turn it back, or I could tell Mom (or Dad)."

3. **"What is the best plan?"**—"I think I'll try asking my sister to turn it back."

4. **"Do the plan"**—"I'll say 'Please turn the show back because I wasn't done watching it.'"

5. **"Did the plan work?"**—"I said it, and my sister turned the TV back to my show."

At first a younger child may need **parental instruction** and even advice when learning and practicing the basic social problem-solving steps. For example, you could give the child advice and ask him or her to try a solution (e.g., "I think you should ask Michelle to turn it back to the channel that you had it on"). This direct instruction approach will still teach the younger child about social problem solving, and if you repeat it frequently, the child will gradually get better at it. Eventually you can use guiding questions, as described in the next section.

Advanced Social Problem Solving for an Older Child or Teen

Review the **Advanced Social Problem Solving** chart at the end of this chapter. This social problem-solving sequence includes two additional steps designed to broaden the child's social problem awareness and incorporates "consequential thinking" into step 5. Discuss an example to show how to use each social problem-solving step, as shown in the chart. Let's say the example is **"Suppose Michael takes my calculator, which makes me mad."**

1. **"Stop! What is the social problem?"**—"Michael took my calculator, which made me mad because I needed it for school, and then I yelled at him."

2. **"Who or what caused the social problem?"**—"Michael took my calculator, but I also got mad and yelled at him."

3. **"What does each person think and feel?"**—"Maybe he felt stressed because he needed a calculator and couldn't find his, but I felt angry because he took it without asking and I needed it."

4. **"What are some plans?"**—"I could hit him, I could ask him to return it and ask to borrow it next time, or I could take something of his."

5. **"Which plan is the most likely to work?"**—"If I hit him, he will probably hit me back and it will make the situation worse. If I ask him to return it and to borrow it next time, he will return it and know what I expect in the future. If I take something of his, I will be doing it to get back at him, and this may lead to more conflict between us. I think I'll try asking him to return it and to borrow it next time."

6. **"Do the plan"**—"I'll say 'You need to return the calculator now and ask to borrow it next time because I may need it.'"

7. **"Did the plan work?"**—"I said it. Michael returned the calculator and apologized."

An older child or teen can profit from **parental guidance** to learn the advanced social problem-solving steps. Here are some suggestions for how the parent might guide the advanced problem-solving process for each step:

1. **Stop! What is the social problem?** *Parent guidance questions: How do you recognize the problem? What is the most accurate way to say what is going on here?*

2. **Who or what caused the social problem?** *Parent guidance questions: It takes two people to have a social problem, right? What is your role, and what is the other person's role in causing this social problem?*

3. **What does each person think and feel?** *Parent guidance questions: What is it like being in the "other guy's shoes," and how does that person think and feel about this social problem?*

4. **What are some plans?** *Parent guidance statements: List as many plans or solutions as possible that could be used to solve the social problem. Don't evaluate them until you think of some possibilities.*

5. **Which plan is the most likely to work?** *Parent guidance questions: Think ahead: What would be the consequences for each plan you just thought of? What would likely happen if you used each of those plans? Which plan will work best?*

6. **Do the plan.** *Parent guidance questions: How will you use the plan? What will you do to make the plan work?*

7. **Did the plan work?** *Parent guidance questions: How did it turn out? (Or: How do you think it will turn out?) What happened? (Or: What will likely happen?)*

This parental guidance approach will teach the older child or teen about social problem-solving steps at a deep level because he or she is doing a lot of active thinking. If you keep doing this, your child will gradually be able to use advanced social problem solving independently. Eventually you can use more guiding questions, like those described in Step 2 below.

PRACTICE EXERCISE

Ask your child to verbally solve other social problems using basic or advanced social problem solving. For a younger child, problems might center on wanting to watch a different TV show than a brother, wanting to play a different game than a visiting friend, or what to do if two children won't let him or her join in a game at recess. For an older child or teen, problems might involve wanting to use a computer being used by a sister, wanting to go to a differ-

BE A ROLE MODEL FOR SOCIAL PROBLEM SOLVING

You can also teach your child by showing how you solve social problems every day. For example, talk out loud about daily or normal situations, such as family members deciding what to make for dinner or how to juggle a demanding schedule of family activities while using basic or advanced social problem solving. Social problem solving can also be demonstrated in an informal way by thinking through situations and problems out loud for your child to observe. For example, when confronted with a social problem, you could say something like, "Hmm, I wonder what the problem is here? What should I do? I think I will try [a strategy/plan]. Did it work?"

ent party than a friend, or what to do if another child or teen spreads a rumor about him or her at school. Consider providing a small reward to your child for practicing this.

Step 2: Coaching Social Problem Solving in Real Life

Help your child apply social problem-solving skills in real-life situations. For example, if your child complains about not being able to get along with a friend, don't suggest what to do; instead prompt him or her to use the social problem-solving steps to figure it out.

Option 1: Informally Reviewing and Dialoguing about Social Problem Solving

The basic or advanced social problem-solving chart can be used to guide a child in the use of social problem solving when real-life problems emerge. Have the child look at the chart and go through the steps. Be sure to guide the child, but don't do the work for him or her! This can be accomplished through *directed discovery,* where you ask guiding questions. For a younger child or an older child who gets stuck, the limited-choice method could be used. However, most children benefit from pondering open-ended questions.

Examples of Limited-Choice Questions

- "You could try this [state option 1] or that [state option 2]." "What do you think would work best?"

- "It looks like you have two options, this [state option 1] or that [state option 2]. "What do you think is the best option?"

Examples of Open-Ended Questions

- "What can you do?"

- "I am confused. Explain it to me. How could you solve that problem?"

- "What are you thinking about to solve that problem?"

- "What's the first step? Then what do you do next? Okay, now what should you do?"

THE IMPORTANCE OF SOCIAL BEHAVIOR SKILLS

You may be able to get your child to come up with a good solution to a social problem, but that doesn't mean he or she will actually use it! For example, a child might solve a social problem for which the solution "I'll ignore her" (if the social problem was being teased) or "Let's take turns" (if the social problem was two people wanting to watch different shows on the same TV). That doesn't necessarily lead to the child's actually doing what was decided. You may need to coach your child on how to follow through. See Chapter 8 for ideas that will help you teach a child social behavior skills. The combination of social behavior and social problem-solving skills can result in the most progress.

Option 2: Formally Reviewing the Advanced Social Problem-Solving Steps

The ***Advanced Social Problem-Solving Worksheet*** at the end of this chapter can be used as a more structured way to guide an older child or teen. Ask your child to answer all questions on the worksheet as he or she solves a social problem. You can still assist by asking limited-choice or open-ended questions, like those above.

PRACTICE EXERCISE
Take some of the examples that were verbally reviewed in the practice exercise for Step 1. Now the idea is to do some role playing to solve those problems using basic or advanced social problem solving. You could act as another child while your child acts as him- or herself. Consider providing a small reward to your child for practicing this.

Consider providing a small reward to your child for using basic or advanced social problem-solving steps with real-life social problems (e.g., use social problem solving seven times to earn a new CD).

Step 3: Use Social Problem Solving to Mediate Sibling Conflict (If Applicable)

A certain amount of sibling conflict is normal and even necessary as children learn to work out their differences. But if siblings have a history of being unable to work out their differences, sibling mediation can help. This is a two-step process: **First**

tell the siblings to separate and cool down for a few minutes. Then bring them together to solve the social problem.

In sibling mediation the child and his or her sibling is guided to use social problem solving to resolve a conflict. When a sibling conflict comes up, try these techniques:

- Sit at a table with you at the head and the siblings on your left and right.

- Tell them that if they commit "fouls," such as name calling, blaming, yelling, or interrupting, the mediation will stop for 5 minutes so they can cool down again before restarting the process.

- Present either the basic or advanced social problem-solving sequence to the siblings.

- Direct them to take turns speaking and go through the social problem-solving steps.

- Keep at it as long as the siblings remain calm and until the issue at hand is resolved.

If in the end the issue cannot be resolved by their efforts, you must resolve it for them (tell them how it is going to be). You may need to use the sibling mediation procedure many times before it starts to work.

PRACTICE EXERCISE

It is a good idea to simulate a sibling mediation session before actually using one to solve a real-life sibling conflict. Make up a sibling dispute and go through a "dry run" of the preceding steps. Consider providing a small reward to the siblings for practicing this.

TROUBLESHOOTING TIP

Sometimes a child just wants his or her way and does not engage in sibling mediation in good faith. The child may even be aggressive to get his or her way. In cases like this it can also help to have a house rule, such as "Siblings must work out their problems in a fair and peaceful way." The combination of such a house rule and peer mediation can be effective in resolving ongoing sibling conflicts. See Chapter 5 for more information on establishing house rules.

Strategy 2: Creating Social Opportunities for Your Child

To learn and practice social problem-solving skills, a child must have the opportunity to interact with peers. **Sometimes a child is neglected (ignored) or rejected (rebuffed) by peers, in which case you may need to assist the child in creating opportunities to be with other children.** With younger children this may occur by arranging play dates. With older children and teens it may mean orchestrating a sleepover, inviting others over for dinner, weekend camping trips, etc. It is best to start with dyads or small groups and perhaps have a certain amount of adult involvement or supervision. **You could plan how the child will work on social problem-solving goals prior to the activity and process how well it went afterward.**

Achieving Success with Social Problem Solving

Social problem solving involves working through disagreements to keep friends and get along better with siblings. This chapter provides ideas and strategies for you to teach and guide your child to develop the ability to recognize and solve social problems. To follow through, periodically review the *Parent Checklist for Child Social Problem Solving* form at the end of this chapter or set your own goals to attain with the *Parenting Goals* form at the end of Chapter 3. It is also a good idea to encourage your child to set specific social problem-solving goals ("Use social problem solving with friends," or "Work on solving problems with my brother [or sister]," etc.) and monitor progress on the *Personal Goals (Basic* or *Advanced)* form at the end of Chapter 3. Consider providing rewards to your child for trying the new social behavior skills (see Chapter 3 for more ideas on motivating your child).

Since social problem solving is somewhat of an advanced skill requiring a certain amount of sophistication, it can take a while to see progress. You need to be **persistent** and **consistent** (i.e., PERCON) in applying these skills-building strategies every day until they work. Sometimes this takes weeks or months.

Parent Checklist for Child Social Problem Solving

Name: _____ Date: _____

In the blanks below, indicate a score for **how well** you make use of that parenting behavior at this time.

	Not too well	**Okay**	**Very well**
	1	2	3

Parent's Efforts in Teaching Child Social Problem-Solving Skills

A. ____ Discussing and practicing social problem-solving skills by reviewing and role-play practicing of social problem-solving steps

B. ____ Coaching social problem solving in "real life" by using questions and dialoguing and/or social problem-solving charts to periodically guide the process

C. ____ Using social problem solving to resolve sibling conflict (if applicable) by acting as a mediator to guide siblings to use this process to work it out

Parent's Efforts in Creating Social Opportunities for the Child

D. ____ Arranging and orchestrating social activities to give the child social opportunities

E. ____ Planning social problem-solving goals prior to the activity and processing how well it went afterward

Basic Social Problem Solving

1. Stop! What is the social problem?

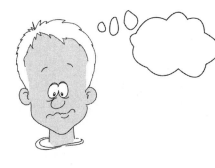

2. What are some plans?

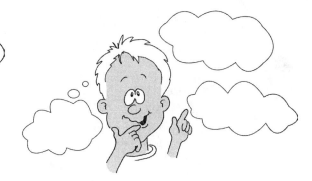

3. What is the best plan?

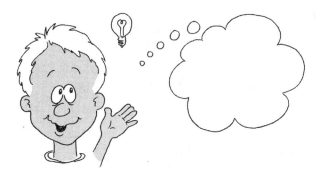

4. Do the plan.

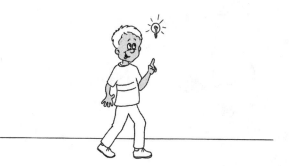

5. Did the plan work?

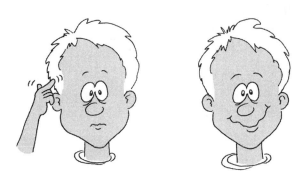

Basic Social Problem Solving

1. **Stop! What is the social problem?**

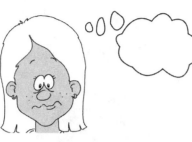

2. **What are some plans?**

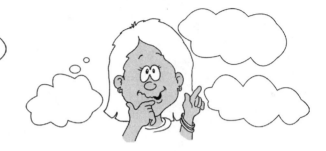

3. **What is the best plan?**

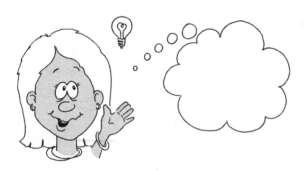

4. **Do the plan.**

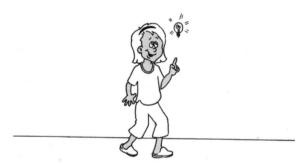

5. **Did the plan work?**

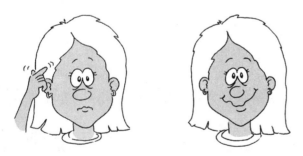

Advanced Social Problem Solving

1. **Stop! What is the social problem?**

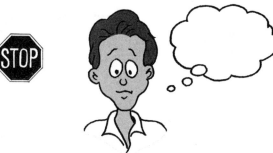

2. **Who or what caused the social problem?**

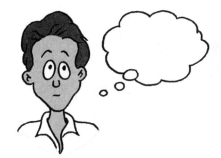

3. **What does each person think and feel?**

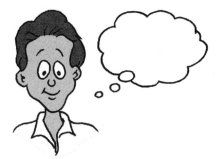

4. **What are some plans?**

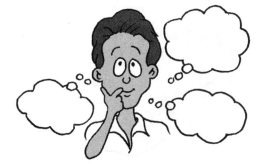

5. **Which plan is the most likely to work?**

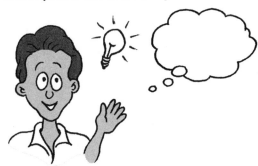

6. **Do the plan.**

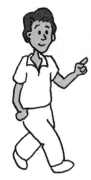

7. **Did the plan work?**

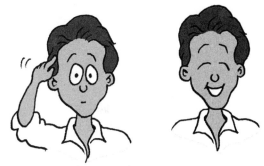

Advanced Social Problem Solving

1. **Stop! What is the social problem?**

 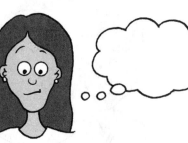

2. **Who or what caused the social problem?**

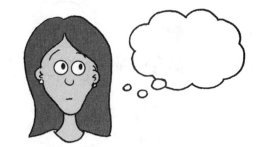

3. **What does each person think and feel?**

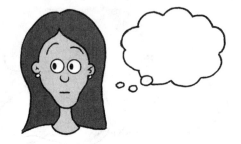

4. **What are some plans?**

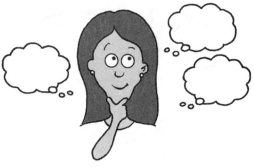

5. **Which plan is the most likely to work?**

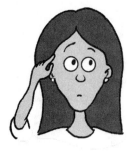

6. **Do the plan.**

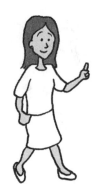

7. **Did the plan work?**

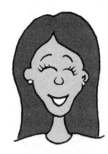

Advanced Social Problem-Solving Worksheet

Name: _____ **Date:** _____

A child/teen and/or parent can complete this worksheet. It's best to fill out the worksheet while you are having a social problem, but it's also okay to fill it out afterward.

1. **Stop! What is the social problem?**

2. **Who or what caused the social problem?** Try to figure out your role and other people's roles in causing the social problem.

3. **What does each person think and feel?** Put yourself in the "other guy's shoes" to see how that person thinks and feels.

4. **What are some plans?** List as many plans or solutions as possible that could be used to solve the social problem.

5. **Which plan is the most likely to work?** Think ahead about what would happen if you used the plans above. Then decide which one will work best.

6. **Do the plan.** How will I do the plan? What will I do to make the plan work?

7. **Did the plan work?**

How Well Did It Work?
(Circle *1*, *2*, *3*, or *4*.)
1. I didn't really try too hard.
2. I sort of tried, but it didn't really work.
3. I tried hard, and it kind of worked.
4. I tried really hard, and it really worked.

10

That Hurts!

Helping Your Child with Bullies

A child who is bullied often endures **physical aggression,** such as hitting and shoving; **verbal abuse,** including teasing, gossip, and insults; **intimidation,** taking the form of glares, gestures, and threats; and **social exclusion,** like being kept out of a group or spreading rumors that isolate the child. Bullying can take place in front of a group of peers who watch or assist the bully or in isolation, such as a one-to-one interaction or in cyberspace. Bullying usually involves a power imbalance where the "victim" is defenseless and controlled by the bully, often being tormented over and over. Typically the bully is a child at school or in the neighborhood, but occasionally it can be a sibling. Bullying can have a significant negative toll on the victims, who sometimes show signs of emotional difficulties, stress, and academic decline. Needless to say, a victim of bullying can use some assistance. This chapter provides ideas for assisting a child who might be the victim of bullying.

Choosing a Focus for Bullies

Start by using the *Parent Checklist for Bullying* (at the end of this chapter) to pinpoint where you are now and focus on what needs work. This checklist will also provide an overview of the topics covered in this chapter. You can refer to the checklist periodically for reminders and to measure your progress.

Strategy 1: Adult Monitoring and Intervention Plan for Your Child

It is absolutely essential that parents, teachers, and other adults get involved with a child who is being bullied. Some adults may disagree, believing that children "need to stand up for themselves." It's unrealistic to expect a child who is being victimized by a bully to go it alone. Remember, children end up bullied because the bully has some kind of power over them. They need adult help and support.

The basic idea is for adults to monitor the situation and set limits on the bully. It is crucial, however, to get your child on board with the idea because the victim needs to tell adults whenever bullying occurs. It may also be a good idea to have a meeting with all adults concerned to plan how to best monitor and set limits.

Here are some ideas for what adults can do to reduce bullying of your child:

- Parents, teachers, and other adults need to be vigilant in watching for instances of bullying and intervene whenever they occur.

- Your child should be encouraged to tell parents, teachers, and other adults about bullying incidents whenever they occur.

- Parents, teachers, and other adults should communicate regularly via phone, e-mail, or notes about how your child is doing at school and whether anyone has witnessed a bullying incident.

- Adults in positions of authority need to talk to the bully and/or provide consequences for bullying behavior. The individuals in authority can also talk to the parents of the bully to state clearly that bullying will not be permitted and to put a concrete plan into action.

It all boils down to the adults being observant, coordinating with one another, and not tolerating bullying behavior. This approach can greatly reduce your child's vulnerability to bullying.

 TROUBLESHOOTING TIP

Children are often reluctant to report occurrences of bullying because they fear retaliation. Reassure your child that reporting bullying is similar to an adult going to the police when threatened by someone. In this case, however,

MAKING AN ENTIRE SCHOOL BUILDING BULLY FREE

Some schools have a schoolwide "bully prevention program," where staff in the entire building monitor hallways, playgrounds, locker rooms, and other areas and enforce a "no tolerance" rule in the classroom and throughout the school. This approach illustrates the general thinking on this topic that it is necessary to get as many adults involved as possible to minimize bullying.

it is the adults who will act like the police. Emphasize that it will be uncomfortable at first but that this will help reduce the problem in the long run and that you will be there for support.

Strategy 2: Teaching Your Child Bully-Coping Skills

The child-focused strategies in this section work best if the adult-focused strategies above are already in place. I don't recommend using these child-focused strategies alone.

As mentioned initially in this chapter, it is tough for a child to stand up to a bully because of the power difference. Nonetheless your child can be taught some behaviors that can at least give him or her a better chance when dealing with the bully.

Step 1: Teaching the "Turtle Technique," or Ignoring Strategy

Make sure your child understands that what keeps a bully going is the victim's reaction and that the bully intimidates to make your child nervous, sad, and/or angry. The bullying is reinforced when your child reacts in this manner, which keeps the bully coming back for more.

One way to cope is to ignore the bully. This can be framed as the "Turtle Technique" for a younger child or as the "ignoring strategy" for an older child or teen. Regardless of age, the imagery of the turtle might help in teaching your child to ignore.

The Turtle Technique, or ignoring strategy, involves not reacting to the bully. Ask your child what would happen if someone tapped a turtle on the shell. He or she more than likely knows that the turtle quickly withdraws into the safety of its shell. Explain that your child can also "be a turtle," or can ignore, whenever the bully strikes. The Turtle Technique, or ignoring strategy, involves:

- Avoiding eye contact.

- Turning away.

- Keeping quiet.

- Thinking "coping thoughts" (e.g., "Don't let him/her bug me," "I'm going to be okay," "I'll try to ignore him").

Next demonstrate what the Turtle Technique, or ignoring strategy, looks like and then do some role play/practice together by taking turns and acting it out.

 PRACTICE EXERCISE
Go over past episodes of bullying with your child. Demonstrate using the Turtle Technique, or ignoring strategy, in that situation, and then have your child practice it with the same situation. Keep this up until your child completely understands and is able to physically perform the Turtle Technique or ignoring strategy.

Coach your child in actually using the Turtle Technique, or ignoring strategy, in bullying situations. This can be accomplished by periodically reminding him or her to do so. You could say something like "Remember to do the Turtle or ignore if [the bully] bothers you today." Check in with your child on a regular basis as to how he or she is dealing with the bully.

Step 2: Teaching the "Courageous Lion Technique," or Assertiveness Strategy

Help your child understand that being prepared and confident will make it possible to take action when dealing with a bully. Your child needs to understand that the bully uses intimidation and enjoys the child's passive acceptance of it. Again, the bullying is reinforced and the bully keeps coming back for more when the child responds in a passive manner to the bully's actions.

One way to cope is to be assertive with the bully. This can be framed as the "Courageous Lion Technique" for a younger child or as the "assertiveness strategy" for an older child or teen. Regardless of age, the image of the lion might help in teaching your child to be assertive.

The Courageous Lion Technique, or assertiveness strategy, involves sticking up for yourself when the bully comes around. Just like the lion in *The Wizard of Oz*, the child can muster up courage and not let the bully get the best of him or her. It should be noted that this technique may not work for some children and depends a lot on the doggedness and threat level of the bully. Use this technique cautiously, because if not done right it could backfire and actually provoke the bully.

The main idea is to respond to the bully by being assertive. "Assertiveness training" is designed to help a child develop and use certain **"say and do"** behaviors to cope with a bully. Ask your child to think ahead and plan what to say and do when confronted by the bully. For example:

- A younger child may plan to say, "Stop bothering me or I will tell the teacher," and then walk into a classroom when being bullied at school.

- A younger child may plan to say, "I have to go home," and then walk home when being bullied in the neighborhood.

- An older child or teen may plan to say, "Knock it off," and then walk into the school building when being bullied in the school parking lot.

- An older child or teen may plan to say, "Leave me alone," and then walk away when being bullied at a school football game.

Next demonstrate what the Courageous Lion Technique, or assertiveness strategy, looks like and then do some role play/practice together by taking turns and acting it out.

USING COMEBACK LINES

The comeback method is related to being assertive and should probably be used only with children who have a fair amount of confidence. It involves using comeback statements designed to take the wind out of the bully's sails. The bully teases, insults, or otherwise antagonizes your child, and then your child says something like:

- "I don't care what you think or say."
- "Are you done yet?"
- "Oh, you again."
- "What have you got to say today [acting uninterested]?"
- "That was a good one."
- "Do you have any more?"
- "What you are saying doesn't bother me."
- "You are entitled to your opinion."

This is only a partial list of comebacks. Many more are possible. The idea is to write down a list of comebacks for your child to say to the bully and then rehearse them via role playing.

Caution your child about comebacks, however. Often they can disarm the bully. Now and then, however, comebacks can incite the bully to do more bullying. Make sure you ask your child how it went and make adjustments if needed.

PRACTICE EXERCISE
Role playing is a good way to rehearse the Courageous Lion Technique, or assertiveness strategy. This involves you and your child acting out various bullying scenarios like the ones above or other situations that are specific to your child. Keep this up until your child completely understands and is able to "perform" the say and do behaviors for handling specific bullying situations.

Coach your child in actually using the Courageous Lion Technique, or assertiveness strategy, in bullying situations. This can be accomplished by periodically reminding him or her to do so. You could say something like "Remember what you will **say and do** if [the bully] bothers you today." Check in with your child on a regular basis as to how he or she is dealing with the bully.

Step 3: Teaching Stress Management Skills

There is some research showing that youth who are bullied experience a lot of stress. Although it won't make the bully stop, learning to express feelings and reduce stress may help your child cope better. You could teach your child stress-coping skills like those described in Chapter 14.

Achieving Success with Bullies

Helping a child with bullies involves working together with your child to figure out ways to reduce bullying directed at him or her. This chapter provides ideas and strategies for you to stop the bullying yourself and to teach and guide your child in using bully-coping behaviors. To follow through, periodically review the *Parent Checklist for Bullying* at the end of this chapter or set your own goals to attain with the *Parenting Goals* form at the end of Chapter 3.

It is also a good idea to encourage your child to set specific bully-coping goals ("I will use Turtle Technique when kids call me names," "Try to be assertive with say and do behaviors if kids bother me at school," etc.) and monitor progress on the *Personal Goals (Basic* or *Advanced)* form at the end of Chapter 3. Consider providing rewards to your child for trying the new bully-coping skills (see Chapter 3 for more ideas on motivating your child).

It can take a lot of effort to organize adults in efforts to stop bullying, and teaching/coaching your child in the best ways to respond to bullying also takes time and effort. You need to be *persistent* and *consistent* (i.e., PERCON) in applying these skills-building strategies every day until they work. Sometimes this takes weeks or months.

Parent Checklist for Bullying

Name: _____ Date: _____

In the blanks below, indicate a score for **how well** you make use of that parenting behavior at this time.

Not too well	Okay	Very well
1	2	3

Parent's Efforts in Adult Monitoring/Intervention Plan

A. _____ Taking steps to help adults be observant, coordinate with each other, and not tolerate bullying behavior toward the child

Parent's Efforts in Teaching the Child to Ignore Bullies

B. _____ Explaining, demonstrating, and role-playing/practicing how to ignore bullies

C. _____ Coaching the child and periodically reviewing how it's going

Parent's Efforts in Teaching the Child to Be Assertive with Bullies

D. _____ Explaining, demonstrating, and role-playing/practicing with the child how to be assertive with bullies

E. _____ Coaching the child and periodically reviewing how it's going

11

Hanging with the "Right Crowd"

Influencing Your Child's Peer Relationships

Research shows that a child's participation in risky behavior and degree of emotional difficulties is greatly influenced by the peers with whom the child spends a lot of time. Associating with troublemaking or troubled peers increases the likelihood that a child will behave similarly. Peer influence can be direct (e.g., peers saying something like "Come on, let's drink some beer") or indirect (e.g., being at a party where everyone is drinking beer). In either scenario a child will feel pressure to conform to the group (i.e., drink beer). The peer influence pattern can be seen as early as preschool and can persist or worsen during the elementary school and teen years. In contrast, a child who is doing well more often than not is associating with other positively developing peers and is involved in constructive activities.

None of this means that your child's friends are necessarily to blame for your child's problems. Parents often get themselves in trouble by labeling their child's friends as "bad" and characterizing their own child as an innocent victim of excessive peer pressure. Demonizing a child's friends often drives a wedge between parent and child and weakens their bond in a way that compromises the ability to build skills together. It's rarely as simple as one child being innocent and another the opposite. The old saying that "birds of a feather flock together" is, in fact, valid. For a variety of reasons, children with similar problems seem to seek each other out, and the negative influence usually goes both ways. It is sometimes challenging to steer a child toward positive peers.

This chapter is for parents who are concerned about their child's friends. It will give you ideas for ways to reduce the impact of your child's affiliation with "negative-influence peers" and promote relationships with "positive-influence peers." The strategies in this chapter, coupled with teaching your child social skills (like those in Chapters 8 and 9), should increase your child's positive peer relationships.

> ### BE PREPARED IF YOUR CHILD DOES NOT WANT TO WORK ON PEER RELATIONSHIPS
>
> Sometimes a child sees no need to discuss or make changes regarding any potentially risky peers he or she hangs out with. If this happens, you need to minimize the potentially negative impact of some of those peer affiliations using Strategy 1 below (things a parent can do) and continue ongoing dialogue with your child about his or her friendships. At some later point your child may be ready to work on positive peer relationships, and then Strategy 2 below (things a child can do) could be a focus.

Choosing a Focus for Peer Relationships

Start by using the *Parent Checklist for Peer Relationships* (at the end of this chapter) to pinpoint where you are now and focus on what needs work. This checklist will also provide an overview of the topics covered in this chapter. You can refer to the same checklist periodically for reminders and to measure your progress.

Strategy 1: Monitoring and Directing Your Child's Peer Contacts

Some degree of peer pressure is a part of nearly every child's daily life. This is especially true nowadays, because most children are connected electronically via social networking and cell phones. It is really hard for children to escape peer pressure and to deal with it! Therefore it is essential for parents to get involved (but not be intrusive) in their child's social lives.

Building a Relationship

Your child is more likely to confide in and work with you on friendship issues if you two have a good relationship. Also, monitoring and directing your child's activities is much more effective when your child trusts your positive motives and has not learned to avoid your scrutiny. Make an extra effort to establish a rapport with your child and repair the bond between you if it is currently weak. Try to spend more quality time together and become more involved in your child's life and activities. Your investment in building a relationship will pay off in increasing your child's desire and inclination to work with you (see Chapter 19 for more ideas for parent–child bonding activities).

Getting to Know Them

It is wise to get to know your child's friends and their parents. Talk to your child's friends and find out about their interests. Open up your home and welcome them. If possible, get to know the parents of the friends and coordinate efforts in keeping track of them.

Monitoring and Supervising

It is typically not a good idea to outright restrict your child from his or her friends except in extreme circumstances where the child's safety is at stake. Instead it is advisable to set some boundaries and limits that diminish any potential negative influence. When your child goes out, always discuss the "four W's." The four W's provide limits regarding social activities and promote a clear understanding between you and your child as to:

- **W**here your child is going

- **W**hom your child is with

- **W**hat your child is doing

- **W**hen your child is coming home

It is also important to monitor what your child is doing on the Internet (social networking sites, chat rooms, etc.) and on his or her cell phone. These personal communication venues provide opportunity for misuse because they are hard to supervise. Have clearly stated rules and expectations about Internet and cell phone usage and frequently check on how your child is using them. It is a good idea to restrict computer and cell phone use in a child's bedroom and late at night because it might be tempting to violate rules regarding usage. Many Internet and cell phone companies now provide parental controls that are worth investigating.

A few extra monitoring pointers may be useful when it comes to preventing drug and alcohol use in an older child or teen. It is no surprise that one of the biggest predictors of a child or teen's substance use is whether the child's peers use! It is noteworthy that most users do so with friends and that most users obtain substances from peers they associate with and/or at parties they attend. Therefore in addition to the four W's:

- Be around on weekends (when substance usage is higher) to monitor your child closely.

- Make sure your child goes only to homes where supervising adults are present and periodically follow up by obtaining parents' home phone numbers and giving them a call.

- Tell your child that you will be available to provide a ride home if the child ends up in an unsupervised setting with substance use occurring (and guaranteeing no questions asked works best).

- Wait up to make sure that your child comes home sober. Look your child in the eye and talk to him or her. Ask about what he or she was doing and about any drug/alcohol use among peers in the places where the child was that night.

- Provide consequences for use even if you think it is only experimentation.

Some parents might be prone to "look the other way" when it comes to their child's substance use. That could be a mistake. Be sure to intervene even if it is only a "gut feeling," because more often than not your gut is correct!

Also be sure to keep the lines of communication open. Talk about your rules and values and provide education about potential harmful effects of substance use and abuse.

 TROUBLESHOOTING TIP

Occasionally a child will be so immersed in a negative peer group that he or she will sneak to hang out with them. If this is a recurring problem, it may be necessary to use the house rules procedure described in Chapter 5. A house rule might be "Parents must know the four W's when you are not home" and/or "Only go to homes in which parents are present." Then privileges are removed when such house rules are violated (see Chapter 5 for details).

Getting Your Child Involved in Positive Organizations

It is a good idea to promote opportunities for interaction with positive-influence peers and adults. Steer your child toward spending time in programs and hanging out at places that provide structured and goal-oriented activities with sufficient adult supervision. These settings might include, but are not limited to, churches, community centers, schools, and park and recreation boards. In these settings your child can get involved in Scouts, sports, after-school programs, arts, theater, dance and music programming, volunteer work, cultural activities, and religious activities, to name a few. These places, and the activities that occur within them, usually have a positive peer culture. Youth then have the opportunity to form friendships with positive-influence peers and can learn from interacting with positive peer and adult role models.

Strategy 2: Teaching Your Child Peer Pressure Coping Skills

This section describes several effective, but difficult to use, peer pressure coping skills. **The child-focused strategies in this section work best if the adult-focused strategies above are in place.** In addition, these are considered to be "advanced" social skills, and therefore the child and parent might benefit from consulting a practitioner.

As mentioned initially in this chapter, standing up to peer pressure is tough. Nonetheless your child can be taught some behaviors that can at least give him or her a better chance when facing it. **Your child will successfully acquire these skills, however, only if the desire and motivation are there.** Several family meetings might be needed to broach the topic and problem-solve about peer pressure (see Chapter 3 for ideas on a family teamwork approach and family meetings). The strategies listed below assume that your child is open-minded and motivated to work on peer pressure.

Discussing Peer Pressure with Your Child

Begin by describing peer pressure and how it can influence your child. It is useful to discuss peer pressure and all of its forms as laid out in the opening paragraph of this chapter. Suggest that the peer pressure might be obvious, such as being encouraged to do something wrong, or subtle, such as peers acting like a "herd" and all doing the wrong thing together. Provide examples such as the following:

- Not knowing what to do when with several peers who suggest they all tease another child on the playground (for child)

- Not knowing what to do when several peers suggest that they all skip school and sneak to the mall, or go to someone's house where there are no adults present, or go to a party where alcohol is available (for older child or teen)

- Not knowing what to do when several peers are discussing how terrible their lives are and how they sometimes think about dying (for older child or teen)

It is also important to help your child understand that pressure can be felt even when the peers don't say anything. For example:

- Explain that if he or she is with a group that is teasing another child, he or she will feel indirect pressure to participate in the teasing because everyone else is doing it (for child).

- Explain that if he or she ends up at a drinking party, the child will feel indirect pressure to drink because everyone else is doing it (for older child or teen).

- Explain that being with people who are dwelling on their personal problems can exert indirect pressure to talk about the child's own problems, which could make him or her feel worse (for older child or teen).

It's important to continue discussing this issue until your child understands what peer pressure is and perhaps at least is entertaining the possibility of figuring out ways to cope with it.

Guiding Your Child in Making Decisions about Peer Pressure

Try to get your child's point of view on the topic of peer pressure and see if he or she is prepared to make some changes. In essence, you want to help your child in making a decision as to whether or not he or she wants to work on peer pressure. Such a discussion may be emotionally charged, so try to stay calm and be supportive. It can also be complicated for a younger child to understand, so it is important to keep it simple.

Help your child talk about his or her experiences of peer pressure and guide a decision process. Perhaps ask about situations in which your child felt pressured by peers and maybe did something he or she later regretted. It might be helpful to announce that "the statute of limitations" has run out, and your child won't get in trouble for sharing things you didn't know about. Ask about peer pressure at school, online, in the neighborhood, etc.

It might be helpful to state that you do not expect your child to drop friends, but you do expect him or her to make good decisions about friends and take action when potentially risky or unsafe situations arise. Guide your child to think about which friends have a positive influence and which friends do not. Ask if your child would like to work on the issue of making good decisions and taking action with peer pressure.

One decision to consider is whether your child might want to broaden his or her circle of friends. Ask your child if he or she might consider contacting old (positive-influence) friends who have fallen by the wayside, reaching out to possible new friends, joining new clubs/organizations, etc.

Some of the methods described in Chapter 3 about assisting your child in setting personal goals, getting motivated, and coming up with a plan could be used with the peer pressure issue, especially with an older child or teen. You could discuss the stages of change or perhaps even guide the child to complete the ***Thinking about Personal Goals*** form as it pertains to a goal of working on peer pressure (at the end of Chapter 3). Once your child makes a decision to work on it, you can brainstorm ideas for dealing with peer pressure and for also cultivating new friendships.

It's important to continue discussing peer relationships until your child decides that he or she wants to work on it. Once that is accomplished, you can work with your child to learn the rest of the skills in this section.

Teaching Your Child Peer Pressure Avoidance Skills

It is really important for your child to understand that one of the best ways to handle peer pressure is to avoid it whenever possible. Do some brainstorming to compile a list of activities and situations in which peer pressure might occur. For younger children, this might include the playground, the neighborhood, or a certain friend's home. For an older child or teen, this might include some of the same situations and being in certain places in the school building, hanging out at the mall, going to unsupervised parties, Internet social networking activities, etc. Help your child understand that these are situations where the child might be influenced directly or indirectly to "do the wrong thing."

Now discuss ways in which your child can avoid the peer pressure situations on the list. Brainstorm to come up with a second list of peer-pressure-dodging techniques. These could include:

- Organizing a group of friends to participate in a positive activity on a weekend night.

- Making excuses for not going to a high-risk event ("My mom won't let me," "I already have plans to . . . ," etc.).

- Ignoring Internet social networking queries.

- Turning off the computer and/or cell phone after a certain hour.

The list of possible peer-pressure-dodging strategies is endless. The more you can think of, the better prepared your child will be for the variety of situations that can arise. Review the peer-pressure-dodging list from time to time to see what you could add to it and how well your child is using the strategies on the list.

Teaching Your Child Peer Pressure Assertiveness Skills

Peer pressure assertiveness skills involve learning to confidently negotiate and manage situations of peer pressure that emerge in the moment. Peer pressure assertiveness is designed to help your child learn to use certain **"say and do"** behaviors. Ask your child to think ahead and plan what to say and do the next time he or she feels pressured to do something wrong. For example:

- A child may plan to say, "No thanks, I have to go home," and then walk home when peers pressure him or her to go into a convenience store to steal candy.

- A child may plan to say, "I don't want to do that," and then walk into the school building when peers pressure him or her to make fun of, or tease, another child on the playground.

- A teen may plan to say, "No thanks, I have to go home," and then go home when peers pressure him or her to go to a party.

- A teen may plan to say, "I don't want to do that," and then walk into the school building when peers pressure him or her to skip school in the school parking lot.

Role playing is a very important tool for learning and practicing the peer pressure assertiveness skills. This involves you and your child acting out various peer pressure scenarios, like the ones described above or other situations that are specific to your child. Go over episodes when your child felt peer pressure. Demonstrate using peer pressure assertiveness skills in that situation and then have your child practice them with the same situation. Keep this up until your child completely understands and can physically perform the peer pressure assertiveness strategy.

Support and coach your child in actually using assertive *say and do* behaviors in peer pressure situations. Remind your child of what to do just before he or she goes out. You could say something like "Remember what you will **say and do** if [a certain peer pressure situation] comes up." Check in with your child on a regular basis as to how it's going with handling peer pressure.

Teaching Your Child Other Social Skills

There is some research showing that children who are rejected (e.g., teased, ostracized, ignored) are more susceptible to negative peer pressure. They are more likely to associate with other rejected children and then are prone to engage in troublemaking behavior. A child who is more socially capable should be less likely to be rejected.

Children with poor social skills are more likely to end up rejected by positive-influence peers because they bug, annoy, hit, and spread rumors, etc., which is not a good way to win friends and influence people! You can teach your child social behavior and social problem-solving skills like those described in Chapters 8 and 9.

Achieving Success with Peer Relationships

This chapter provides ideas and strategies with which you can lessen the impact of negative-influence peers and promote your child's involvement with positive-influence peers. To follow through, periodically review the **_Parent Checklist for Peer Relationships_** at the end of this chapter or set your own goals to attain with the **_Parenting Goals_** form at the end of Chapter 3. It is also a good idea to encourage your child to set specific peer-pressure-coping goals ("Stay away from park after dark to avoid getting in trouble," "Turn off Facebook and cell phone after 8 P.M. each night," "Use assertive say and do strategies when asked to do things that I really don't want to do," etc.) and monitor progress on the **_Personal Goals (Basic_** or **_Advanced)_** form at the end of Chapter 3. Consider providing rewards to your child for trying the new peer-pressure-coping skills (see Chapter 3 for more ideas on motivating your child).

The peer group means so much to children and especially teens. It will undoubtedly take a fair amount of effort to address this issue if it is a major concern. You need to be **persistent** and **consistent** (i.e., PERCON) in applying these skills-building strategies every day until they work. Sometimes this takes weeks or months.

Parent Checklist for Peer Relationships

Name: _____ **Date:** _____

In the blanks below, indicate a score for how well you make use of that parenting behavior at this time.

Not too well	Okay	Very well
1	2	3

Parent's Efforts in Monitoring and Directing Peer Contacts

A. _____ Making an extra effort to establish a rapport and bond with the child to enhance the child's willingness to work on positive peer relationships

B. _____ Getting to know the child's friends and their parents

C. _____ Knowing the four W's when child is out and monitoring Internet and cell phone use

D. _____ Checking up on the child to prevent drug use

E. _____ Getting the child involved in programs and places that provide positive structured activities with adult supervision

Parent's Efforts in Teaching the Child Peer Pressure Coping Skills

F. _____ Discussing peer pressure with the child

G. _____ Helping the child make decisions to work on dealing with peer pressure

H. _____ Discussing and brainstorming ideas and techniques that the child can use to avoid peer pressure situations

I. _____ Explaining, demonstrating, and role-playing/practicing methods that the child can use to respond assertively to peer pressure situations

J. _____ Coaching the child and periodically reviewing how well he or she is dealing with peer pressure

Enhancing Your Child's Emotional Development

12 Let It Out!

Teaching Your Child to Understand
and Express Feelings

We all know it can be difficult to handle negative or uncomfortable feelings. This
is especially true for a child. Yet keeping harmful feelings all bottled up inside can
take a toll. A child who does this may act out angry, anxious, and/or sad feelings by
way of problem behaviors, or those feelings may fester until the child develops serious emotional problems. This chapter provides ideas and techniques for teaching
your child about feelings and how to express them in a healthy way.

Choosing a Focus for Feelings

Start by using the *Parent Checklist for Child Feelings* (at the end of this chapter) to
pinpoint where you are now and focus on what needs work. This checklist will also
provide an overview of the topic covered in this chapter. You can refer to the checklist periodically for reminders and to measure your progress.

Strategy 1: Teaching Your Child to Understand Feelings

There are two feelings charts in this chapter that can be used to educate your child
about emotions and words to describe them. The *Basic Feelings Vocabulary Chart*
(at the end of this chapter) shows pictures of feelings and words that are appropriate for a younger child. The *Advanced Feelings Vocabulary Chart* (at the end of
this chapter) shows many more pictures of feelings and words that are appropriate

for an older child or teen. Use the one that you think matches your child's stage of emotional development.

- Show the chosen chart to your child.

- Ask if your child understands the words for the feelings on the chart.

- Work together to define the words (a children's or standard dictionary can help).

- Ask if your child has experienced any of those feelings and when they occurred.

- Talk about times when you may have experienced any of those feelings yourself.

It's important to explain the words for the feelings clearly so that your child understands each feeling. Keep reviewing the chart, perhaps over several days, until you are sure that your child knows and understands most of the words for the feelings.

PRACTICE EXERCISES

It can be fun and informative to make faces to match the chart. Take turns making the faces and see if each of you can match that expression with the one on the chart.

With younger children, a version of the "Simon says" game is fun. Take turns playing Simon. Simon names a feeling (e.g., "frustrated"), and then the other person acts out the feeling (e.g., being and looking frustrated).

Take turns discussing past events when you or your child had certain feelings on the chart. Start with positive events and feelings to get this going. For example, you could say that someone at work complimented you for a task you accomplished, which made you feel proud and joyful. Then go to some of the negative events and feelings if it is going well. For example, your child could discuss feeling hurt and sad when someone called him or her a name. Help your child understand the connection between events in life and feelings.

It's important for your child to know that negative and positive feelings are a natural reaction to what is going on in our lives. Explain to a younger child that life has its up and down moments and that our feelings go up and down too. An older child or teen might benefit from knowing that feelings are "signals" that tell us how

---

PERSPECTIVE TAKING

Perspective taking is really important in getting along with others. One important part of perspective taking is to recognize others' feelings. Consider discussing all of the feelings that have been reviewed as they relate to others. Guide your child to think of others' feelings. This could be as simple as wondering about the feelings of characters in a book or a movie. Or it could be discussing the feelings of family members as events unfold that day. You could use the **Basic** or **Advanced Feelings Vocabulary Chart** as a reference for discussing the feelings of others.

---

the daily events we experience are affecting us. If we listen to those signals, we can get better at dealing with the feelings we are experiencing.

It can also be useful for an older child or teen to understand how feelings can be affected by our thoughts and behaviors. The *Feelings, Thoughts, and Behaviors Go Together* chart (at the end of this chapter) shows that unhelpful thoughts and unhelpful behaviors are related to negative feelings, whereas helpful thoughts and helpful behaviors are related to positive feelings. Explain that thoughts are internal ways in which we talk to ourselves, and behaviors are the actions we take in everyday life. Note that some of our thoughts and feelings are unhelpful or not good for us, whereas others are helpful or good for us. Go through the examples on the chart to show how feelings, thoughts, and behaviors are related. Share real-life examples and then ask your child for real-life examples that demonstrate how these go together in a manner similar to what is depicted on the chart.

The take-home message is that understanding our feelings and how they affect us can lead us to do something to prevent our feelings from getting the better of us. In other words, tell your child that although we cannot make our feelings just go away, we can manage them. This can be accomplished by expressing feelings (the topic of this chapter) or by changing our thinking and behaving (the topics of Chapters 13 and 14, respectively). Note that the goal here is to focus on feelings and that thoughts and behaviors will be touched on later.

 PRACTICE EXERCISE
Revisit the examples that came up in the preceding practice exercise. Take turns discussing past events, but this time also review related thoughts and feelings that came up and discuss how they were connected. Start with positive events and then go to negative.

Strategy 2: Teaching Your Child to Express Feelings

Suggest to your child that *"getting our feelings out"* can help us feel better. For a younger child the balloon analogy can be useful. Ask what happens when you keep blowing up a balloon. It eventually stretches to the point where it pops. Keeping all of your feelings inside is similar. They eventually build up and can pop out (or overwhelm us). Explain to your child, for example, that if someone hurts his or her feelings by teasing him or her, and your child keeps these feelings inside, the feelings might build up to sadness or anger that can pop out (by crying or shouting). Suggest further that talking about his or her feelings may not make the problems go away, but it can make your child feel better by getting them out.

With an older child or teen the same teasing example could be discussed but perhaps without the balloon analogy. The older child or teen can be told that letting feelings build up can be overwhelming at times. Note that although talking about feelings does not solve life's problems, this can be an effective way to cope or deal with them.

Tell your child that the lesson here is that **it is important to understand and express feelings.**

Informally Reviewing and Dialoguing about Feelings

Ask your child to calm down and then discuss feelings on the **Basic or Advanced Feelings Vocabulary Chart** to understand and express feelings at that moment with your assistance. Be sure to guide your child, but don't express the feelings for him or her! Instead ask guiding questions—a method called "directed discovery." For example, for a child who was ignored by a classmate at school that day, you could:

- Ask limited-choice questions, such as "Are you sad or hurt or both?"

- Ask open-ended questions, such as "What are you feeling right now?"

- Label feelings, such as stating "You look sad and hurt."

For most children open-ended questions will elicit an expression of what the child felt. When a child gets stuck and can't quite label a feeling, you could then try limited-choice questions or labeling to give the child possibilities to consider.

Look for opportunities to discuss and label your child's feelings as events unfold. Be sure to notice, comment, and praise your child for expressing feelings.

MODELING HOW TO EXPRESS FEELINGS

Try to be aware of times when you are experiencing feelings and express them each day. Practice expressing these feelings so that your child can observe you. For example, if you accidentally drop and break your cell phone, you could get out the **Basic** or **Advanced Feelings Vocabulary Chart** and point to the feeling "frustrated" and then state "That makes me feel frustrated!"

Formally Reviewing and Dialoguing about Feelings Using a Diary

The **Feelings Diary** form (at the end of this chapter) can also be used by your child to write down positive and negative events that occur in a day and different feelings that go along with these events.

- Guide your child to fill out the diary.

- Act as the "secretary" who writes down what the child says in the diary.

- Give your child the option of sharing the diary or keeping it private.

You might consider providing a small reward to your child for completing the **Feelings Diary** (e.g., five diaries could earn a trip to the cinema).

Many children also benefit when parents fill out a **Feelings Diary** and shares it with them. This helps the child feel less alone in the process and gives the child the added benefit of learning by observing you. If you decide to keep a **Feelings Diary** too, be sure to write about neutral and not-too-personal events. For example, it would be helpful to write about how you felt in a traffic jam, but not how you felt while arguing with your spouse or partner.

Achieving Success with Feelings

Feelings skills involve identifying and expressing feelings with friends and family. This chapter provides ideas and strategies to help you promote your child's awareness of his or her feelings and how to express them. To follow through, periodically review the **Parent Checklist for Child Feelings** form at the end of this chapter or set your own goals to attain with the **Parenting Goals** form at the end of Chapter 3. It is also a good idea to encourage your child to set specific feelings goals (e.g., "Fill out the *Feelings Diary* for a week," "Be open to discussing things going on in my life and how I feel," etc.) and monitor progress on the *Personal Goals (Basic* or *Advanced)* form at the end of Chapter 3. Consider providing rewards to your child for trying the new feelings skills (see Chapter 3 for more ideas on motivating your child).

Some children are uncomfortable with their feelings and are reluctant to express them. You need to be **persistent** and **consistent** (i.e., PERCON) in applying these skills-building strategies every day until they work. Sometimes this takes weeks or months.

Parent Checklist for Child Feelings

Name: _____ **Date:** _____

In the blanks below, indicate a score for **how well** you make use of that parenting behavior at this time.

Not too well	Okay	Very well
1	2	3

Parent's Efforts in Teaching Child Feelings Skills

A. _____ Reviewing feelings-oriented chart(s) to educate the child about different feelings and words to describe them

B. _____ Teaching the child about how feelings are related to thoughts and behaviors

C. _____ Using informal discussion and/or feelings charts to periodically guide feelings expression

D. _____ Being a good role model about how to express feelings

Basic Feelings Vocabulary Chart

Afraid

Happy

Lonely

Mad

Sad

Surprised

Advanced Feelings Vocabulary Chart

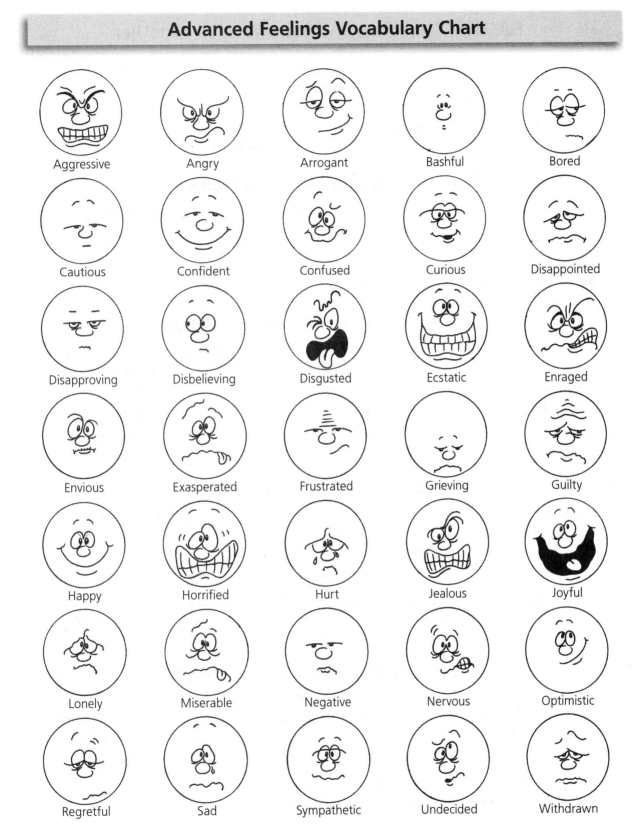

Aggressive	Angry	Arrogant	Bashful	Bored
Cautious	Confident	Confused	Curious	Disappointed
Disapproving	Disbelieving	Disgusted	Ecstatic	Enraged
Envious	Exasperated	Frustrated	Grieving	Guilty
Happy	Horrified	Hurt	Jealous	Joyful
Lonely	Miserable	Negative	Nervous	Optimistic
Regretful	Sad	Sympathetic	Undecided	Withdrawn

Feelings, Thoughts, and Behaviors Go Together

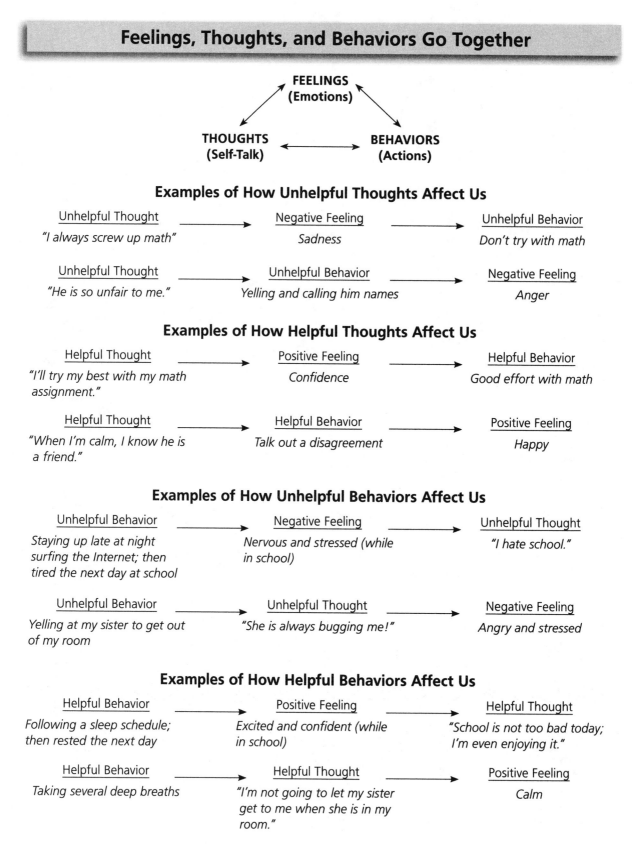

FEELINGS
(Emotions)

THOUGHTS
(Self-Talk)

BEHAVIORS
(Actions)

Examples of How Unhelpful Thoughts Affect Us

Unhelpful Thought → Negative Feeling → Unhelpful Behavior

"I always screw up math" — *Sadness* — *Don't try with math*

Unhelpful Thought → Unhelpful Behavior → Negative Feeling

"He is so unfair to me." — *Yelling and calling him names* — *Anger*

Examples of How Helpful Thoughts Affect Us

Helpful Thought → Positive Feeling → Helpful Behavior

"I'll try my best with my math assignment." — *Confidence* — *Good effort with math*

Helpful Thought → Helpful Behavior → Positive Feeling

"When I'm calm, I know he is a friend." — *Talk out a disagreement* — *Happy*

Examples of How Unhelpful Behaviors Affect Us

Unhelpful Behavior → Negative Feeling → Unhelpful Thought

Staying up late at night surfing the Internet; then tired the next day at school — *Nervous and stressed (while in school)* — *"I hate school."*

Unhelpful Behavior → Unhelpful Thought → Negative Feeling

Yelling at my sister to get out of my room — *"She is always bugging me!"* — *Angry and stressed*

Examples of How Helpful Behaviors Affect Us

Helpful Behavior → Positive Feeling → Helpful Thought

Following a sleep schedule; then rested the next day — *Excited and confident (while in school)* — *"School is not too bad today; I'm even enjoying it."*

Helpful Behavior → Helpful Thought → Positive Feeling

Taking several deep breaths — *"I'm not going to let my sister get to me when she is in my room."* — *Calm*

Feelings Diary

Name: _____ **Date:** _____

Write down positive and negative events that happened and how you felt. Use the (**Basic** or **Advanced**) **Feelings Vocabulary Chart** to help label your feelings. You can fill the diary out when an event occurs or afterward. You can share this **Feelings Diary** with others or keep it private.

Positive Events	**My Feelings**
1.	1.
2.	2.
3.	3.
4.	4.

Negative Events	**My Feelings**
1.	1.
2.	2.
3.	3.
4.	4.

13

You Are What You Think

Teaching Your Child to Think Helpful Thoughts

Unfortunately some children think unhelpful thoughts, which can negatively affect their feelings and behavior. Unhelpful thoughts in children typically fall into three categories:

- **Worry thoughts:** Some children tend to expect the worst or at least think something bad is going to happen. Worried thinking is often associated with feeling nervous and can lead to avoidant behavior.

- **Downer thoughts:** Some children think that things are bad and nothing can make them better. Downer thinking is often related to feeling sad and can lead to withdrawn behavior.

- **Unfriendly thoughts:** Some children think people are unfair and doing mean things to them on purpose. Unfriendly thoughts are often related to feeling angry and can lead to aggressive or defiant behavior.

A child who often has thoughts in these categories may need assistance in developing a more helpful way of thinking. This chapter provides ideas for helping your child to start thinking more helpful thoughts so that he or she can feel and behave better.

Choosing a Focus for Helpful Thinking

Start by using the *Parent Checklist for Child Helpful Thoughts* (at the end of this chapter) to pinpoint where you are now and focus on what needs work. This checklist will also provide an overview of the topics covered in this chapter. You can refer to the checklist periodically for reminders and to measure your progress.

Strategy 1: Promoting Awareness of Thinking in Your Child

TROUBLESHOOTING TIP

The ideas and procedures in this section are most relevant to an older child or teen who has the ability to think somewhat abstractly. The goal is to increase awareness in your child of how thoughts affect him or her every day. If you think the ideas here are "over the head" of your child, just skip to "Basic Helpful Thoughts for a Younger Child" under the second strategy. Use your judgment about whether your child will understand the ideas presented here.

Step 1: Helping Your Child Understand Thoughts

The *Feelings, Thoughts, and Behaviors Go Together* chart at the end of Chapter 12 shows how thoughts influence one's feelings and behaviors. It is recommended that you go back to the chart and review it until your child "sees" these connections. It is important for your child to understand that he or she can try to have helpful thoughts, which can then impact feelings and behaviors in a positive or helpful way.

Step 2: Identifying How Your Child Tends to Think

The *Unhelpful Thoughts List* (at the end of this chapter) can be used to help your child understand what type of unhelpful thoughts he or she tends to have and the effects of such thinking. With a younger child it may be better to review this verbally and informally, but an older child or teen could fill out the form. Use your child's responses to dialogue about his or her unhelpful thoughts. Ask the child to identify which type of unhelpful thoughts he or she has most often.

Explain to your child that many of these unhelpful thoughts are sometimes referred to as **A**utomatic **N**egative **T**houghts, or "ANTs." Say that it is good idea to be aware of these ANTs during normal everyday activities because they may lead to problems if left unchecked.

Next, review the *Helpful Thoughts List* (at the end of this chapter) to help your child understand the effects of helpful thoughts. Again, with a younger child it may be better to review this verbally and informally, but an older child or teen could read it and discuss the form. Have a conversation with your child to discuss the benefits of helpful thoughts. **The primary goal is for your child to recognize how helpful thoughts are related to more positive feelings and helpful actions.** Ask your child to identify which type of helpful thoughts he or she should work on the most.

Explain that when unhelpful thoughts, or ANTs, pop up, your child can change course and have more helpful thoughts. In the process your child will have more positive feelings and helpful behavior.

Strategy 2: Teaching Your Child to Think Helpful Thoughts

Step 1: Instructing Your Child about Helpful Thought Skills

Now that your child is more aware of being able to learn to change thinking patterns, you can use one of two different sequences of helpful thought steps that follow: basic or advanced. These lists will be useful for children and teens at different stages of development.

Basic Helpful Thoughts for a Younger Child

Review the **Basic Helpful Thoughts** chart (at the end of this chapter). Discuss an example of using helpful thoughts and go through each step as shown in the chart. Let's say the example is **"I am having a hard time doing a math worksheet and I think, 'Boy, I am stupid—this is way too hard for me'"**:

1. **"Am I thinking unhelpful thoughts?"**—"Yes, I am. I am thinking of myself as stupid."

2. **"Are these thoughts going to help me?"**—"No. This thinking will make me feel like giving up."

3. **"What is a different and more helpful way I can think?"**—"I know I am smart in many school subjects, but math is hard. I just need to keep at it or ask for help."

At first a younger child may need **parental instruction** in the basic helpful thinking steps. You can ask the three questions above, but if the child gets stuck you could give him or her some possible answers (like those depicted above). You could give the child advice and ask him or her to try it (e.g., "It might be best to think 'I am smart in many school subjects, but math is hard. I just need to keep at it or ask for help'"). This direct instruction approach will still teach the younger child about helpful thinking, and if you repeat it a lot, your child will gradually get better and better at it. Eventually you can use more coaching questions like those described in the next section.

Advanced Helpful Thoughts for an Older Child or Teen

Review the ***Advanced Helpful Thoughts*** chart (at the end of this chapter). Discuss an example of using helpful thoughts and go through each step as shown in the chart. Let's say the example is **"I am in a hallway at school, and Melissa doesn't look at me and walks right by. Then I think, 'She is avoiding me on purpose. I guess she doesn't like me anymore'"**:

1. **"Am I thinking unhelpful thoughts?"**—"Yes, I am. I am thinking that Melissa is being mean and doesn't like me."

2. **"What kind of unhelpful thoughts am I having?"**—"Those are Unfriendly and Downer Thoughts."

3. **"How are these unhelpful thoughts going to make me feel and act?"**—"I feel angry, lonely, and sad. It makes me want to tell her off and then stay away from her."

4. **"What is a different and more helpful way I can think?"**—"Maybe Melissa didn't see me. She probably does like me, because we do sometimes hang out. Maybe I am jumping to conclusions."

5. **"What kind of helpful thoughts am I having?"**—"Those are Friendly and Upper Thoughts."

6. **"How are these helpful thoughts going to make me feel and act?"**—"Calmer and more hopeful. I will make an effort to say 'hi' to Melissa the next time I see her."

An older child or teen can profit from **parental guidance** to learn the advanced helpful thinking steps. Here are some suggestions for how you might guide the advanced helpful thinking process for each step:

1. **Am I thinking unhelpful thoughts?** *Parent guidance questions: Are you having unhelpful thoughts right now? What are these unhelpful thoughts? How do you recognize whether your thoughts are unhelpful?*

2. **What kind of unhelpful thoughts am I having?** *Parent guidance questions: There are different kinds of unhelpful thoughts, right? What kind of unhelpful thoughts are you having? Are your unhelpful thoughts Worry, Downer, or Unfriendly?*

3. **How are these unhelpful thoughts going to make me feel and act?** *Parent*

guidance questions: What negative feelings will you have if you keep thinking the unhelpful thoughts? What actions might you take, or how might you behave, if you keep thinking the unhelpful thoughts?

4. **What is a different and more helpful way I can think?** *Parent guidance questions: How else can you think about this that might be more helpful? What helpful counterthoughts can you use to replace the unhelpful thoughts?*

5. **What kind of helpful thoughts am I having?** *Parent guidance question: Are your helpful counterthoughts Confidence, Upper, or Friendly?*

6. **How are these helpful thoughts going to make me feel and act?** *Parent guidance questions: What positive feelings will you have if you keep thinking the helpful thoughts? What actions might you take or how might you behave if you keep thinking the helpful thoughts?*

This parental guidance approach will teach the older child or teen about helpful thinking at a deep level, because he or she is doing a lot of active thinking. If you keep doing this, your child will gradually be able to use advanced helpful thinking independently. Eventually you can use more coaching questions, like those described in Step 2 below.

 PRACTICE EXERCISE
Ask your child to think about situations where basic or advanced helpful thoughts could be used. For a younger child, helpful thoughts might be used when someone on the playground ignores the child or when a teacher reprimands him or her for talking. For an older child or teen, helpful thinking might be used when he or she hears of a party but has not been invited or when a parent reprimands the child for not doing chores. In these examples, ask your child to go through either basic or advanced helpful thought steps.

MODEL HELPFUL THINKING

You can also teach your child by modeling helpful thinking. Talk out loud when you have unhelpful thoughts and then show how you changed the thoughts to make them more helpful. For example, you forget an appointment and think "I must be going senile. I can't remember anything." Demonstrate using basic or advanced helpful thought steps while your child observes.

Step 2: Coaching Your Child in Helpful Thoughts

The next task is to teach your child to change unhelpful thoughts to more helpful ones in the moment. When you notice that your child is saying things out loud that reflect unhelpful thoughts, it may be a good idea to guide him or her in this process.

Option 1: Informally Reviewing and Dialoguing about Helpful Thoughts

Ask your child to calm down and then go through the steps on the **Basic** or **Advanced Helpful Thoughts** chart to examine and change thinking at that moment with your assistance. Be sure to guide your child, but don't do the thinking for him or her! Instead ask guiding questions—a process called "directed discovery"—that are either open-ended or limited-choice. For a younger child or an older child who gets stuck, the limited-choice method could be used. However, most children benefit from open-ended questions.

Examples of Limited-Choice Questions

- "Is that an unhelpful or helpful way to think?"

- "Are those worry thoughts?"

- "Are you having ANTs right now?"

- "You could think [one example of helpful thoughts] or that [another example of helpful thoughts]."

- "Maybe it would be better to think some confidence thoughts like. . . . "

Examples of Open-Ended Questions

- "Are you thinking unhelpful thoughts?"

- "What is a more helpful way to think?"

- "What type of unhelpful thought is that?"

- "Is that type of thinking going to help you?"

- "Okay, what is a more helpful way to think?"

- "What do you think would be most helpful?"

THE NEED TO "CHILL BEFORE THINKING"

Research and experience inform us that we do not think straight when nervous, angry, agitated, or otherwise upset. It's very important to calm down in order to think in a helpful way. With this in mind, try to help your child calm down so that he or she can think straight. Guide your child to go somewhere for a few minutes to calm down, take a few breaths, etc. See Chapter 14 for more ideas about teaching your child to stay calm.

Be sure to notice, comment, and praise your child for using helpful thoughts. You might even consider providing a small reward for going through the steps on the **Basic** or **Advanced Helpful Thoughts** chart with real life-episodes (e.g., go through the steps five times to earn a trip to the cinema).

Option 2: Formally Reviewing the Unhelpful Thoughts Worksheet

You can also use the **Advanced Helpful Thoughts Worksheet** (at the end of this chapter) to guide an older child or teen through the steps toward helpful thoughts. When you see your child having unhelpful thoughts, ask the child to calm down and then answer all the questions on the worksheet as the child examines and changes his or her thoughts. You can still assist by asking limited-choice or open-ended questions. **Consider providing a small reward to your older child or teen for using the worksheet (e.g., fill out seven worksheets to earn a new CD).**

TROUBLESHOOTING TIP
Some children get defensive when a parent points out that they are having unhelpful thoughts (your child might say "No, I'm not—you are," or "It's your fault"). If this happens, don't push it or it could backfire, with the child getting angry. Maybe bring it up later, when the child is calmer and more receptive. Be sure to be a good role model as a person who cultivates helpful thoughts.

Achieving Success with Helpful Thinking

Learning to increase helpful thoughts involves recognizing unhelpful thoughts and changing them into ones that are more helpful. This chapter provides ideas and strategies for you to promote this important skill for emotional development in your child. To follow through, periodically review the *Parent Checklist for Child Helpful Thoughts* or set your own goals to attain with the *Parenting Goals* form at the end of Chapter 3. It is also a good idea to encourage your child to set specific helpful thinking goals ("Fill out the *Advanced Helpful Thoughts* worksheet once per day for a week," "Cool off when I get upset to clear my head of ANTs," "Review my personal helpful thoughts list each morning before school," etc.) and monitor progress on the *Personal Goals (Basic* or *Advanced)* form at the end of Chapter 3. Consider providing rewards to your child for trying the new helpful thinking skills (see Chapter 3 for more ideas on motivating your child).

The skills presented in this chapter are relatively sophisticated. Sometimes a child is defensive about having unhelpful thoughts. Progress can be made, however, with a lot of effort. You need to be **persistent** and **consistent** (i.e., PERCON) in applying these skills-building strategies every day until they work. Sometimes this takes weeks or months.

Parent Checklist for Child Helpful Thoughts

Name: _____ **Date:** _____

In the blanks below, indicate a score for **how well** you make use of that parenting behavior at this time.

Not too well	**Okay**	**Very well**
1	2	3

Parent's Efforts in Promoting Child's Awareness of Unhelpful and Helpful Thoughts

A. ____ Explaining how unhelpful and helpful thoughts relate to how one feels and behaves so that the child is more aware

Parent's Efforts in Teaching a Child Helpful Thoughts Skills

B. ____ Reviewing and role-playing/practicing of helpful thoughts steps

C. ____ Using informal discussion and/or helpful thoughts charts to periodically guide helpful thoughts skills

D. ____ Modeling helpful thinking

E. ____ Coaching the child to calm down so that thoughts can be more helpful (i.e., "chill before thinking")

Unhelpful Thoughts List

Listed below is a variety of thoughts children may have about themselves. Read each thought and indicate how frequently that thought (or a similar thought) typically occurs for you over an average week. There is no right or wrong answer to these questions. Use the 3-point rating scale to answer how often you have these thoughts:

1	**2**	**3**
Rarely	**Sometimes**	**Often**

Worry Thoughts

1. ____ Something bad will happen to me (family member, friend, teachers, etc.).
2. ____ It will be terrible (horrible, scary, etc.).
3. ____ Everyone will be looking at me, and I won't know what to say.
4. ____ I don't fit in with the crowd.
5. ____ I won't be able to do it.
6. ____ My future doesn't look good. Nothing will work out for me.
7. ____ *My usual worry thoughts are (write in):* _____

_____

Downer Thoughts

8. ____ I'm no good (stupid, ugly, weak, etc.).
9. ____ I can't do anything right (I'm a failure).
10. ____ I have to do well in school, sports, and so forth, or people will look down on me.
11. ____ I give up. I've tried everything. There's nothing more I can do.
12. ____ It's my fault.
13. ____ No one likes me.
14. ____ *My usual downer thoughts are (write in):* _____

_____

Unfriendly Thoughts

15. ____ Lots of peers (siblings) are mean to me on purpose.
16. ____ Lots of peers (siblings) are unfair to me.
17. ____ My parent (teacher) is unfair to me.
18. ____ Lots of peers (siblings) mess with me (tease me, pick on me).
19. ____ My parent (teacher) is to blame.
20. ____ My parent wants to run my life.
21. ____ *My usual unfriendly thoughts are (write in):* _____

_____

For each thought you rated a 3, ask yourself the following questions:

1. How am I going to **feel** if I have this thought?
2. How am I going to **act or behave** if I have this thought?
3. Is this an unhelpful thought that I should be more aware of and try to change?

From *Skills Training for Struggling Kids*. Copyright 2013 by The Guilford Press.

Helpful Thoughts List

Listed below are helpful counterthoughts that children can use instead of unhelpful thoughts. Unhelpful (Worry) Thought #1 corresponds to Helpful (Confidence) Thought #1, and so on. Compare the unhelpful thoughts to the helpful thoughts.

Confidence Thoughts

1. It's not likely that something bad will happen to me (family member, friend, teachers, etc.).
2. It will be all right (just fine, etc.) if I do my best.
3. I am imagining that everyone will be looking at me. I'll know what to say once I get there.
4. I fit in with some people. I do have friends.
5. I can do my best if I try.
6. My future will be fine as long as I do my best.
7. *Other confident thoughts I could think are (write in):* _____

_____

Upper Thoughts

8. I know I have lots of good points. I'm just fine the way I am.
9. I do lots of things quite well, actually.
10. I'll just try my best. People respect others who try.
11. It doesn't help to give up. I need to keep trying.
12. It doesn't help to find fault. I need to think of how to make it better.
13. I have some friends. If I want more, I can do something about that if I try.
14. *Other upper thoughts I could think are (write in):* _____

_____

Friendly Thoughts

15. When I'm calm, I realize that most peers (my siblings) treat me okay.
16. When I'm calm, I realize that most peers (my siblings) are fair to me.
17. When I'm calm, I realize that my parent (teacher) is usually fair to me.
18. Most of the time I get treated okay by peers (siblings).
19. It doesn't help to blame my parent (teacher). I need to think about solutions.
20. My parent is just trying to make sure I am safe and that I do well.
21. *Other friendly thoughts I could think are (write in):* _____

_____

For each counterthought you choose, ask yourself the following questions:

1. How am I going to **feel** if I have this thought?
2. How am I going to **act or behave** if I have this thought?
3. Is this a helpful thought that I should be more aware of and try to keep?

Basic Helpful Thoughts

1. Am I thinking unhelpful thoughts?

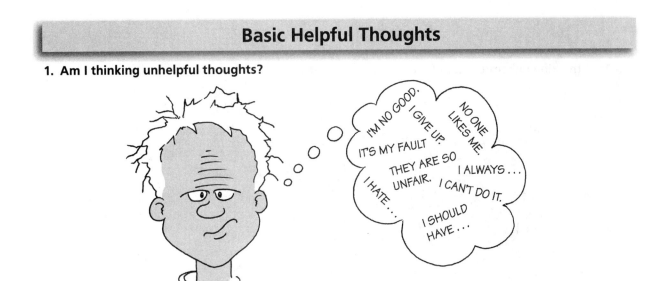

2. Are these thoughts going to help me?

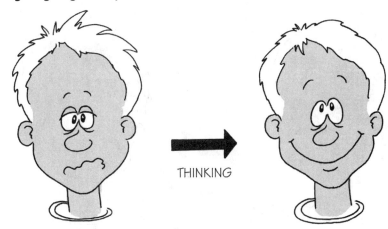

THINKING

3. What is a different and more helpful way I can think?

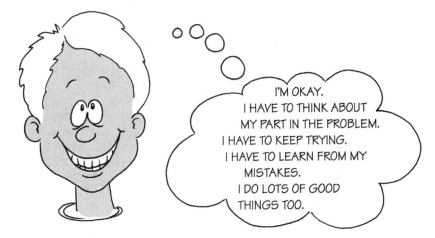

From *Skills Training for Struggling Kids.* Copyright 2013 by The Guilford Press.

Basic Helpful Thoughts

1. Am I thinking unhelpful thoughts?

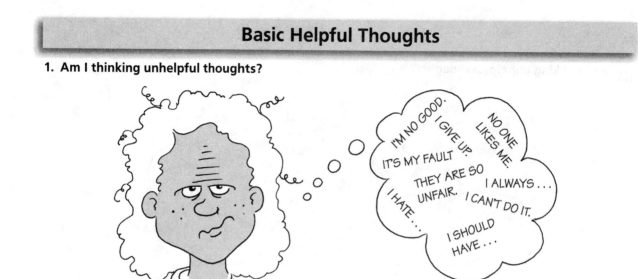

2. Are these thoughts going to help me?

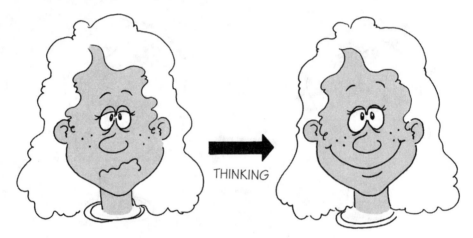

3. What is a different and more helpful way I can think?

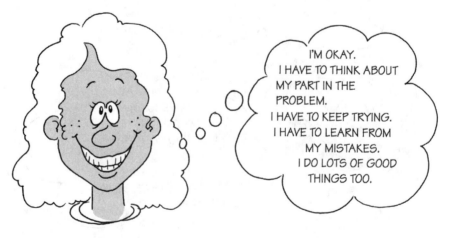

Advanced Helpful Thoughts

1. Am I thinking unhelpful thoughts?

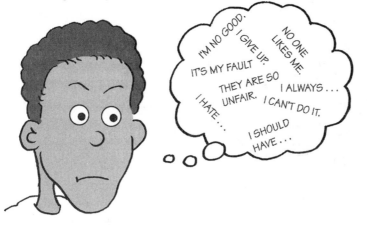

2. What kind of unhelpful thoughts am I having? Are they . . .

- **Worry Thoughts**—like thinking the worst or that something bad will happen?
- **Downer Thoughts**—like things are bad and nothing can make them better?
- **Unfriendly Thoughts**—like people are unfair and doing mean things on purpose?

3. How are these unhelpful thoughts going to make me feel and act?

4. What is a different and more helpful way I can think?

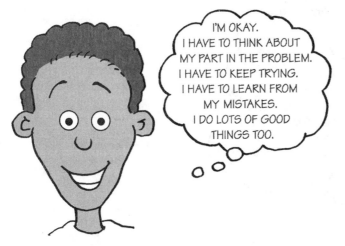

5. What kind of helpful thoughts am I now having? Are they . . .

- **Confidence Thoughts**—like I can handle it if I try?
- **Upper Thoughts**—like I can make them better if I try?
- **Friendly Thoughts**—like most people treat me okay most of the time?

6. How are these helpful thoughts going to make me feel and act?

Advanced Helpful Thoughts

1. Am I thinking unhelpful thoughts?

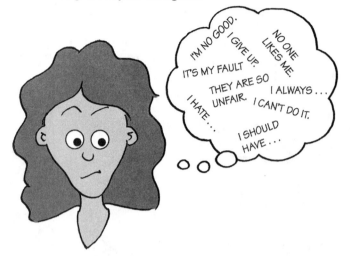

2. What kind of unhelpful thoughts am I having? Are they . . .

- **Worry Thoughts**—like thinking the worst or that something bad will happen?
- **Downer Thoughts**—like things are bad and nothing can make them better?
- **Unfriendly Thoughts**—like people are unfair and doing mean things on purpose?

3. How are these unhelpful thoughts going to make me feel and act?

4. What is a different and more helpful way I can think?

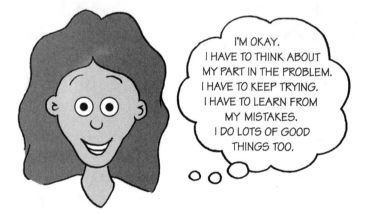

5. What kind of helpful thoughts am I now having? Are they . . .

- **Confidence Thoughts**—like I can handle it if I try?
- **Upper Thoughts**—like I can make them better if I try?
- **Friendly Thoughts**—like most people treat me okay most of the time?

6. How are these helpful thoughts going to make me feel and act?

Advanced Helpful Thoughts Worksheet

Name: _____ **Date:** _____

Fill out the worksheet during or after you have experienced an unhelpful thought.

1. What are my thoughts? Am I thinking unhelpful thoughts?

2. What kind of unhelpful thoughts am I having? Are they (circle those that apply) . . .
- **Worry Thoughts**—like thinking the worst or that something bad will happen?

- **Downer Thoughts**—like things are bad and nothing can make them better?

- **Unfriendly Thoughts**—like people are unfair and doing mean things on purpose?

3. How are these unhelpful thoughts going to make me feel and act?

4. What is a different and more helpful way I can think?

5. What kind of helpful thoughts am I now having? Are they (circle those that apply) . . .
- **Confidence Thoughts**—like I can handle it if I try?

- **Upper Thoughts**—like I can make them better if I try?

- **Friendly Thoughts**—like most people treat me okay most of the time?

6. How are these helpful thoughts going to make me feel and act?

How Well Did It Work?
(Circle *1, 2, 3,* or *4.*)

1. I didn't really try too hard.
2. I sort of tried, but it didn't really work.
3. I tried hard, and it kind of worked.
4. I tried really hard, and it really worked.

14

Stress Busters

Teaching Your Child to Manage Stress

Stress is an emotional and physical arousal response to a problem or challenging situation. Unfortunately, some children have a hard time coping with challenging situations and may display frustration, tension, anger outbursts, and/or nervousness that is out of proportion to the situation. This chapter describes **general stress reduction** and **in-the-moment stress-coping** strategies to help your child learn skills for managing stress that will also reduces episodes of anxiety and anger.

Choosing a Focus for Stress Management

Start by using the *Parent Checklist for Child Stress Management* (at the end of this chapter) to pinpoint where you are now and focus on what needs work. This checklist will also provide an overview of what the topics covered in this chapter are about. You can refer to the checklist periodically for reminders and to measure your progress.

Strategy 1: Promoting Awareness of Stress in Your Child

Many children don't fully understand what stress is or know when they're experiencing it. If your child seems to be among them, you'll get more cooperation with working on managing stress if you start out by explaining that stress occurs when someone feels like an everyday problem is too much to handle and doesn't take helpful action to deal with it. Offer examples with which your child might identify, such as finding schoolwork too hard and therefore avoiding it, or being bugged by a peer and then yelling at the other child.

With an older child or teen you can expand this discussion by reviewing the *Feelings, Thoughts, and Behaviors Go Together* chart that was introduced in Chapter 12 of this book. This chart depicts how unhelpful and helpful behaviors are related to thoughts and feelings that can either increase or reduce stress. Reviewing the chart can help an older child or teen understand that he or she can try to have helpful behaviors, which can impact feelings and thoughts in a positive or helpful way.

After reviewing what stress is, ask if your child gets "stressed out," such as feeling tense or nervous or upset or angry. Ask your child for personal examples, and if he or she cannot come up with examples, you can try tactfully providing some. Examples that could come up include a child who reports that some kids were laughing at her during school and she felt angry, and a child who says that he failed a school assignment and felt nervous knowing that his mother would find out. You might offer some personal examples, such as being behind at work and feeling tense or cooking a big meal for many relatives and how it was stressful. After discussing examples, ask your child if he or she would like to work on better managing or dealing with stress. Explain that you will help.

Strategy 2: Helping Your Child Develop Stress-Reduction Skills

A child's general stress level can be reduced by taking ongoing effective action. This section gives ideas that can buffer stress and help a child feel better.

Promoting Healthy Daily Habits

These commonsense actions are **proactive** ways for keeping general stress at a manageable level. A child might benefit from:

- **Exercising regularly.** Facilitate your child's participation in sports or going for walks, playing outside, or going to a health club with you.

- **Relaxing periodically.** Help your child build in down time for reading, playing a musical instrument, pursuing a hobby, and/or regularly practicing meditation and/or yoga.

- **Getting enough sleep.** Most experts agree that a younger child needs 10 or more hours of sleep per night, and a teen, 8 or more hours. Good sleep habits include having a consistent bedtime, avoiding large meals near bedtime, avoiding "wind-up activities" such as computer/video/TV or exercise just before bed, engaging in "wind-down activities" like reading a book or listening to soft music before bed, etc. It is also a good idea to avoid long naps in the afternoon.

- **Socializing more.** It is universally accepted that socializing with family and positive-influence peers reduces stress. If your child is isolated, try to organize or provide opportunities for him or her to get out more to hang out with family and friends. With younger children this may be accomplished by arranging "play dates." With older children and teens it may mean orchestrating a sleepover, inviting others over for dinner, weekend camping trips, etc.

- **Developing a routine.** At the most basic level, it is a good idea to have relatively consistent times for waking up, eating meals, doing homework, relaxing, playing, and going to bed (see Chapter 19 for more ideas).

- **Keeping up with schoolwork (avoiding procrastination).** Although technically not a health habit, getting behind at school can affect your child's health through all of the stress it causes. Playing catch-up is very hard on everyone involved. Help your child develop good school-related habits and stay with them (see Chapter 15 for more ideas).

Each of these general stress-reduction methods can help a stressed-out child, but it would be overwhelming to try to tackle all of them at the same time, so try to narrow it down. Start with the habit that seems easiest to form. Even the easy ones, however, require action, and your child is most likely to take action consistently if you help him or her set concrete goals, such as using the *Personal Goals* (*Basic* or *Advanced*) form in Chapter 3.

TROUBLESHOOTING TIP

You and your family can have a lot of influence on your child's stress-reduction habits. You too can take action and begin an exercise routine, get on a more consistent schedule, or engage in a favorite hobby. A child who sees a parent exhibiting stress-reduction behaviors may be more inclined to follow suit. Finally, the family can also take action together. Consider making it a team effort to prevent stress and get healthy!

Promoting Behavioral Activation

No doubt you've heard people say: "Don't just sit there; do something!" Sometimes a child can be so overwhelmed with stress and problems that he or she becomes stuck and more or less shuts down. Such inaction often takes the form of (1) avoiding situations or responsibilities, (2) withdrawing or isolating from others, and (3) overthinking (worrying and ruminating) about problems. If any of these shut-down behaviors are typical for your child, then behavioral activation might help.

Behavioral activation focuses primarily on changing behaviors to promote better coping with stress. Behavioral activation involves engaging in activities you value, enjoy, and find rewarding and, in so doing, getting more positive reinforcement into your life. This in turn improves your emotional well-being. Engaging in the stress-reduction strategies noted above is related to behavioral activation in a general sense, but in this section it is applied specifically to avoiding, withdrawing, and/or overthinking (worrying and ruminating).

The first step is to discuss avoiding, withdrawing, and/or overthinking in a way that your child will understand. Mention that everyone has stress but that how you deal with it determines whether it is helpful or not. Note that avoiding, withdrawing, and/or overthinking can be signs that stress is too high and that a person is having a hard time. To make the point, consider reviewing some examples:

- *Avoiding behavior* might be evident in staying away from certain peers, not going to school, procrastinating with homework, not discussing feelings or problems, etc.

- *Withdrawing behavior* might be expressed as sitting in a bedroom a lot, watching too much TV, texting instead of talking to people, etc.

- *Overthinking* could be occurring when a child keeps dwelling on the same problems, worries endlessly about friendships, keeps reviewing past mistakes over and over in his or her mind, etc.

Ask your child if he or she might be feeling stressed out and responding to it with avoiding, withdrawing, and/or overthinking. Consider giving your child some supportive feedback and discussing examples from the past. With an older child or teen you can also elaborate by again reviewing the *Feelings, Thoughts, and Behaviors Go Together* chart (at the end of Chapter 12). It is good to make the connection that avoiding and withdrawing are unproductive behaviors that can affect feelings and thoughts in a negative way and that overthinking involves thoughts that can affect feelings and behaviors in a negative way.

The next step is to help the child to recognize avoiding, withdrawing, and/ or overthinking when it is occurring and then to take action. The child should be encouraged to "stop and take action," including:

- Stop avoiding and take action

- Stop withdrawing and take action

- Stop thinking and take action

The actions to take can include exercising, relaxing with a favorite activity, socializing with friends/family or engaging in some type of helpful goal-directed behavior, such as cleaning one's bedroom, homework, etc. Ask your child to generate a list of specific things he or she can do to take action in response to avoiding, withdrawing, and/or overthinking. Provide some suggestions if your child is open to hearing them.

The **Personal Goals (Basic** or **Advanced)** form (at the end of Chapter 3) can be used to work on behavioral activation. A goal might be to "Stop thinking and go for a walk," "Stop sitting in my room and talk to Mom," "Stop worrying about homework and do it for at least 15 minutes," etc. Parents can encourage or reward follow-through to increase the child's motivation to use behavioral activation (see Chapter 3 for more ideas on motivation).

Strategy 3: Teaching Your Child In-the-Moment Stress-Coping Skills

Every now and then a highly difficult event or situation comes up, and it's critical that children susceptible to stress learn how to cope with intense stress reactions in the moment. **Although these are reactive ways for managing stress, it takes a lot of proactive planning and practicing for a child to be prepared to use them effectively** on the spot. Be forewarned that each step below could take a week or more to accomplish, so you and your child need to be very motivated and willing to put in the effort! (If you need a refresher, go back to Chapter 3 for motivational guidance.)

 TROUBLESHOOTING TIP

Under certain circumstances these stress-coping strategies are not the best way to handle a child's problematic reactions to challenging situations. One is when the child's stress (anger, agitation, etc.) seems to come mainly from not

getting his or her way or having to follow parental rules. This is more likely a behavior problem, in which case it will be more fruitful to work on parenting strategies to improve the child's behavior (see Chapters 4–7). Another is when others in the family get upset at the same time, which may be related more to family conflict than to one child's inability to cope with stress. In that case it may be beneficial to work on family interaction skills (see Chapter 20).

Step 1: Teaching Your Child to Recognize Stress Spikes

It's important for your child to know that stress is one response to daily challenges, and that it's sometimes experienced as feelings of frustration, nervousness, anger, and the like. Sometimes events can be overwhelming, causing stress to spike. Explain to your child that a spike is a sudden, rapid rise in stress that can range from low (mild) to high (very intense). To put coping strategies into effect when needed, your child has to be able to recognize a stress spike. Tell your child that, in the same way that a traffic light signals a driver to take action, there are body signals, thought signals, and behavior signals that indicate high stress and a need for action. These signals are noticeable in a variety of different ways, including:

Body Signals

- Increased breathing
- Increased heart rate
- Increased sweating
- Red face color
- Tense muscles
- Body feels "hot"

Thought Signals

- "I hate you."
- "I can't do it."
- "It will be awful."
- "She is so unfair."
- "You are so stupid."
- "I'm going to hit him."
- "I hate doing homework."
- "They will just ignore me."
- "I want to break something."
- "I am dumb."
- "I can't do anything right."
- "I give up."

Behavior Signals

- Avoid
- Punch/hit
- Threaten
- Faint
- Run
- Withdraw

- Yell
- Cry
- Fidget
- Tremble

Work with your child to write down personal body, thought, and behavior signals for stress spikes to increase awareness. Perhaps you could both recall one or more times when your child was stressed out (couldn't find something needed for school, someone called him or her a name, a sibling grabbed the TV remote without asking, etc.). Generate a list of the body, thought, and behavior signals your child may have experienced during those situations (similar to the signals above).

 PRACTICE EXERCISES

A younger child can have a hard time understanding something inside the body that cannot be seen or touched. To explain body signals, ask your young child to try running in place for 30–60 seconds and then think about how his or her body feels in terms of the body signals above. Explain that the body feels similarly during a stress spike episode and that it is a good idea to be more aware.

Another practice strategy is to help your child keep a simple journal for a week or two, noting events that made him or her upset, nervous, or angry and what the body, thought, or behavior signals were. The younger child will require the help of a parent to keep such a journal, whereas the older child or teen could do it independently if motivated (see Chapter 3 for ideas on promoting a child's motivation).

Step 2: Teaching Your Child Relaxation

Your child can learn to reduce body tension through relaxation, but the best method for teaching the child varies in relation to age. Try the following methods one at a time to see which one works best for your child. Make sure that your child really knows one relaxation skill before practicing another.

Belly (or Diaphragmatic) Breathing

The basic idea behind belly breathing (technically, diaphragmatic breathing) is to inhale and exhale slowly using one's entire lung capacity. Explain to your child that the goal is to breathe, starting from the belly (diaphragm) region of the lungs to the top. **To get this latter point across, ask your child to blow up a balloon. He or she will observe that the bottom of the balloon fills before the top.**

Ask your child to lie down, sit, or stand to practice. Prompt him or her to be comfortable and relaxed and then take breaths using a **slow, low, and through-the-nose** breathing technique:

- **Slow** means take your time. Initially it is a good idea to count slowly to 4 for the exhale, pause or hold your breath to the count of 2 (to avoid getting dizzy), and then count to 4 for the inhale (i.e., "4–2–4 breathing"). Over a few days (or weeks) of practice, gradually strive to make the exhale longer than the inhale by slowly counting to 6, 2, and 4, respectively (i.e., "6–2–4" breathing).

- **Low** means that during the inhale, you fill the lungs at the lowest point first and then move your breath up to the top (like the balloon). For practice, place a hand on the belly (diaphragm) and observe it going up and down.

- **Through the nose** is just that. Keep your mouth shut and breathe only through your nose.

Repeat at least four times and gradually work up to as many times as is comfortable. It's okay to rest between breaths to avoid hyperventilation.

 PRACTICE EXERCISE
It takes time to learn correct belly (diaphragmatic) breathing. Encourage your child to practice each day for 5 or 10 minutes. Consider providing a small reward to your child for practicing this breathing exercise.

Muscle Tension–Release Technique

Ask your young child to tense up all the muscles in his or her body and imagine being a **robot**. Have the child hold this position for approximately 10–15 seconds. Then ask your child to release all the tension and imagine being a **rag doll,** with all muscles very loose, and holding this relaxed state for 10–15 seconds. Repeat several times.

Ask your older child or a teen to tense up and then release small muscle groups one at a time. The idea is to tense up one muscle group (e.g., feet) for 10–15 seconds, then release or relax that muscle group for 10–15 seconds, and then repeat the tension-and-release sequence with different muscle groups, starting from the bottom and moving up. For example, your child would tense and release feet, then lower legs, upper legs, abdomen, chest, shoulders, neck, and finally the face. Afterward the entire body will be relaxed.

PRACTICE EXERCISE
Ask your child to set aside 5 or 10 minutes a day to practice these relaxation techniques. After a few practice episodes, ask the child to try running in place for 30–60 seconds and then use relaxation techniques to calm down. Consider providing a small reward to your child for practicing a relaxation technique.

Visualization

Explain to your child that it helps to "see" (imagine) him- or herself as calm in a high-stress moment. For example, if a peer or a sibling calls your child a name, your child can **imagine** him- or herself remaining calm. Alternatively, ask your child to visualize some sort of barrier that won't let the stress in, like a "force field" or a wall, off which stress bounces. Ask your child to describe his or her own personal visualization that is most relaxing for him or her during stress spike episodes.

Step 3: Teaching Your Child to Use Calming Self-Talk

This next skill involves talking to oneself in a calming manner. Explain to your child that calming self-talk involves saying things to him or her (usually in his or her head, not out loud) to cope with stress. Here are some examples of calming self-talk:

- "Take it easy."
- "Stay cool."
- "Chill out."
- "Take some deep breaths."
- "I'm getting tense, so I need to relax."
- "Don't let him bug me."

- "I'm going to be okay."
- "It's okay if I'm not good at this."
- "I'm sad that Emily doesn't want to hang out with me, but many other people like me."
- "I'll just try my hardest."
- "Try not to give up."

PRACTICE EXERCISE
It can be helpful to rehearse different scenarios and then practice calming self-talk. One scenario might be that a sibling turns the channel on the TV when your child is watching it. Have your child imagine this and then use calming self-talk to cope with it (e.g., "I'm not gonna let this get me upset" or "I'm gonna tell him it made me angry and next time to ask me if it is okay to turn the channel"). Do as many such practices as needed until your child

has the technique down. Consider providing a small reward to your child for practicing calming self-talk.

Step 4: Teaching Your Child to Take Effective Action

The final step in learning how to manage stress is to take action and/or solve the problem that originally caused the stress, anger, nervousness, etc. Taking action might involve going somewhere to cool down for a few minutes (like a bedroom or outdoors), expressing feelings, asking for a hug, being assertive with someone, etc.

 PRACTICE EXERCISE

It can be helpful to rehearse different scenarios and then practice taking effective action. For example, revisit the scenario where your child is watching TV and a sibling turns the channel. Have your child imagine this and then take effective action (e.g., figure out what he or she will say to the sibling, rehearse it, and then say it). Do as many such practices as needed until your child has the technique down. Consider providing a small reward to the child for practicing.

Step 5: Coaching Your Child to Use In-the-Moment Stress-Coping Skills in "Real Life"

After your child develops the skills described above, you can prompt him or her to use some of them or all of them at once when stressed, anxious, upset, or angry.

Option 1: Informally Reviewing and Dialoguing about Staying Calm

Use the **Staying Calm** chart (at the end of this chapter) as a visual guide to help your child (especially the younger child). When stress episodes occur, you can coach your child by prompting and guiding him or her to answer the questions on the chart. Consider providing a small reward to your child for using the **Staying Calm** chart (e.g., go through the chart five times to earn 30 minutes of special time with a parent).

Option 2: Formally Reviewing Staying Calm Worksheet

Use the **Staying Calm Worksheet** (at the end of this chapter) to help an older child or teen through the stress management steps. It is a good idea to assist an older child or teen with a few worksheets and gradually turn over responsibility for completing it to the child. Consider providing a small reward to your older child or teen for completing the worksheet (e.g., fill out seven worksheets to earn a new CD).

Achieving Success with Stress Management

Stress management involves maintaining a healthy lifestyle and being able to calm down when a stressful event occurs. This chapter provides ideas and strategies for helping your child develop these important lifelong skills. To follow through, periodically review the *Parent Checklist for Child Stress Management* at the end of this chapter or set your own goals to attain with the *Parenting Goals* form at the end of Chapter 3. It is also a good idea to encourage your child to set specific stress management goals ("Take dog for a 20-minute walk every day after school and before homework," "Try to stay calm by recognizing body signals and taking deep breaths," etc.) and monitor progress on the *Personal Goals (Basic* or *Advanced)* form at the end of Chapter 3. Consider providing rewards to your child for trying the new stress management skills (see Chapter 3 for more ideas on motivating your child).

This chapter presents many skills, so it's wise to focus on one or two at a time. It is better to be good at a few skills than okay at many of them. In addition, the skills presented in this chapter are perhaps the most difficult in the "Struggling Kids" program. Indeed, many adults are not good at them! This means that a lot of effort will be required. You need to be **persistent** and **consistent** (i.e., PERCON) in applying these skills-building strategies every day until they work. Sometimes this takes weeks or months.

Parent Checklist for Child Stress Management

Name: _____ **Date:** _____

In the blanks below, indicate a score for **how well** you make use of that parenting behavior at this time.

Not too well	Okay	Very well
1	2	3

Parent's Efforts in Promoting Child's Awareness of Stress

A. _____ Explaining what stress is so that the child is more aware

Parent's Efforts in Teaching a Child Stress-Reduction Skills

B. _____ Helping the child develop good habits related to diet, exercising, relaxing, sleeping, etc.

C. _____ Incorporating routines and schedules into everyday life

D. _____ Taking action to follow through with healthy habits

E. _____ Guiding behavioral activation as needed by helping the child recognize ineffective coping and taking action as planned to enhance coping

Parent's Efforts in Teaching a Child In-the-Moment Stress-Coping Skills

F. _____ Educating the child about stress and body, thought, and action "stress signals"

G. _____ Guiding use of breathing, muscle tension–release relaxation, and visualization techniques to relax

H. _____ Guiding use of coping self-talk when stressed out

I. _____ Guiding taking action, like expressing feelings, asking for a hug, going for a walk, relaxing, asserting, etc.

J. _____ Asking guiding questions and/or using charts to prompt the child to use stress management in real life

K. _____ Being a good model for managing stress

Staying Calm

1. What am I stressed, angry, or nervous about?

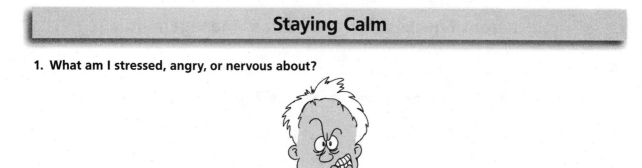

2. How stressed, or angry, or nervous am I?

1	2	3	4	5
Not at all	A little	Somewhat	A lot	Very much

3. Calm down my body with slow breathing, muscle relaxation, and visualization.

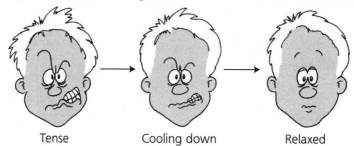

Tense   Cooling down   Relaxed

4. Use calming self-talk.

IT'S OK. I CAN HANDLE THIS.

I'M GOING TO TRY TO RELAX.

I'M NOT GOING TO LET IT GET TO ME!

5. Take some action to solve the problem.

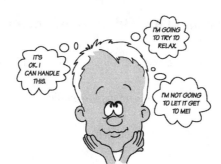

Staying Calm

1. What am I stressed, angry, or nervous about?

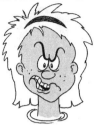

2. How stressed, or angry, or nervous am I?

1	2	3	4	5
Not at all	A little	Somewhat	A lot	Very much

3. Calm down my body with slow breathing, muscle relaxation, and visualization.

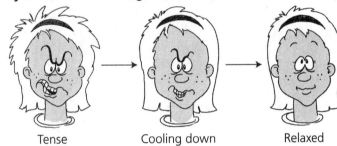

Tense   Cooling down   Relaxed

4. Use calming self-talk.

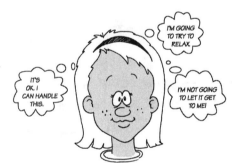

IT'S OK. I CAN HANDLE THIS.

I'M GOING TO TRY TO RELAX.

I'M NOT GOING TO LET IT GET TO ME!

5. Take some action to solve the problem.

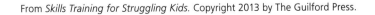

Staying Calm

1. What am I stressed, angry, or nervous about?

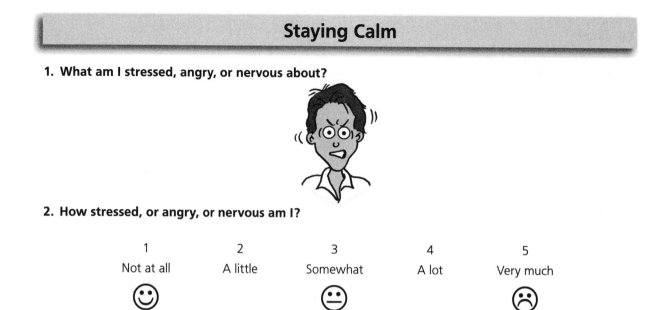

2. How stressed, or angry, or nervous am I?

1	2	3	4	5
Not at all	A little	Somewhat	A lot	Very much

3. Calm down my body with slow breathing, muscle relaxation, and visualization.

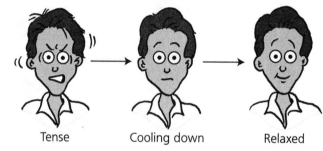

Tense → Cooling down → Relaxed

4. Use calming self-talk.

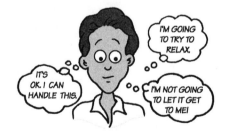

IT'S OK. I CAN HANDLE THIS.

I'M GOING TO TRY TO RELAX.

I'M NOT GOING TO LET IT GET TO ME!

5. Take some action to solve the problem.

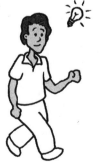

Staying Calm

1. What am I stressed, angry, or nervous about?

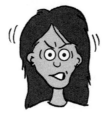

2. How stressed, or angry, or nervous am I?

1	2	3	4	5
Not at all	A little	Somewhat	A lot	Very much

3. Calm down my body with slow breathing, muscle relaxation, and visualization.

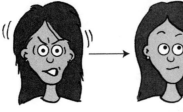

Tense → Cooling down → Relaxed

4. Use calming self-talk.

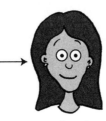

IT'S OK. I CAN HANDLE THIS.

I'M GOING TO TRY TO RELAX.

I'M NOT GOING TO LET IT GET TO ME!

5. Take some action to solve the problem.

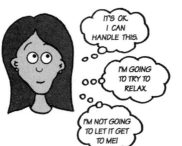

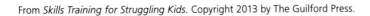

Staying Calm Worksheet

Name: _____ **Date:** _____

A child/teen and/or parent can complete this worksheet. It's best to fill out the worksheet while you are upset, but it's also okay to fill it out afterward.

1. What am I stressed, angry, or nervous about? _____

2. How stressed, angry, or nervous am I? (Circle one.)

1	2	3	4	5
Not at all	A little	Somewhat	A lot	Very much

3. What are the signals that tell me I am stressed out?

   a. **Body signals:**

   b. **Thought signals:**

   c. **Behavior signals:**

4. What can I do to slow my breathing and relax my body?

5. What calming self-talk can I use to cope?

6. What action can I take to deal with the situation or solve the problem?

How Well Did It Work?
(Circle *1, 2, 3,* or *4.*)

1. **I didn't really try too hard.**
2. **I sort of tried, but it didn't really work.**
3. **I tried hard, and it kind of worked.**
4. **I tried really hard, and it really worked.**

Enhancing Your Child's Academic Development

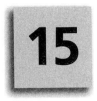

15

Surviving School

Teaching Your Child to Manage Time, Organize, Plan, Review, and Stay on Task

Teachers will tell you that academic achievement is equal parts ability and performance. Performance at school means creating products to show what has been learned, and this is accomplished by completing work. Many children struggle at school because they don't have well-developed learning-related habits or skills. This chapter offers ideas for teaching your child "school survival skills"—managing time, organizing, planning, reviewing, and staying on task. I recommend actively assisting your child in learning these school survival skills so you know that they are ingrained and then gradually turning over responsibility to the child so that he or she can use the skills independently. It is never too early to work on these skills. In fact, you can begin planting the seeds for developing good habits during early elementary school and continue to develop them through the teen years.

 TROUBLESHOOTING TIP
This chapter contains a lot of information! You can't do it all, and you probably don't need to. Children who have the broad category of school performance problems have many different types of struggles—therefore, many ideas are presented. You'll need to pick and choose a few that seem to fit you and your child best and go from there. Consult with your practitioner to help you choose the best methods for your child.

Choosing a Focus for School Survival Skills

Start by using the *Parent Checklist for School Survival Skills* (at the end of this chapter) to pinpoint where you are now and focus on what needs work. This checklist will also provide an overview of the topics covered in this chapter. You can refer to the checklist periodically for reminders and to measure your progress.

Strategy 1: Establishing a Mandatory Homework Time

A mandatory homework time provides a strong foundation for academic success. The goals of mandatory homework are to get things done for school **and** to provide a forum for learning and practicing school survival skills (many of these skills are described in this chapter). Begin by designating a quiet spot for your child to do homework. If you have a child who is prone to get off task, it is helpful for the home-work spot to be within your eyesight so he or she can be monitored. Then assign a (relatively) consistent time on each school night (often Sunday–Thursday) during which your child *must* work the entire time. The general rule is to allow a minimum of 10 minutes for each grade (e.g., 20 minutes for a second grader, 100 minutes for a 10th grader, etc.). Knowing that no exceptions will be made on the duration tells your child that nothing is gained by rushing or by "forgetting" to bring home school materials.

It is a good idea for you and your child to discuss a definition of homework going forward. Most children define homework as getting done what is due tomorrow as fast as possible! Suggest a new definition of homework that focuses on present, future, and past goals. Redefine homework as (1) **getting things done that are due**, (2) **organizing and planning, and** (3) **reviewing.**

Parent involvement is crucial, especially at first. You must provide scaffolding as your child learns new habits. Tell your child that he or she will be required to work with you for part of this time each day. At a minimum it is a good idea to "check in" with the child at the beginning of homework to help the child get organized and "check out" the child at the end of homework to see if everything got done. As your child forms new habits and makes progress, you can gradually fade out and be less involved.

If homework causes stress in your child, then include some basic stress man-agement as part of the mandatory homework procedure. It can helpful to allow your child to relax and maybe get some exercise before homework. In addition, some of the stress management strategies described in Chapter 14 can be considered part of mandatory homework. For example, a stressed-out fifth grader could work on deep breathing and/or rehearsing personalized calming self-talk statements (related to homework) for the first 5 minutes of his 50-minute mandatory homework session. This still leaves 45 minutes for academic homework and hopefully a less stressed child who is doing it! It also teaches your child to stay calm when studying. **Use a**

timer to keep track of the minutes. Allow your child to take breaks, but stop the timer during them and restart it once your child returns. This can be a helpful first step in your child's learning very basic time management skills.

If homework has historically been a struggle for your child, it might be a good idea to reward him or her for doing it for the first few weeks. This helps to establish a routine. For example, he or she could earn a new DVD or a special activity after successfully completing 10 sessions of mandatory homework time.

Mandatory homework time also affords your child an opportunity to learn and practice many of the skills described below. Select strategies that you think would be helpful to your child and use them during this time (see later section for details).

TROUBLESHOOTING TIP
The most common difficulty with mandatory homework time is that the parent or the child (or both) gets frustrated. Remember that you are in the lead in this activity and your mood will influence your child's. Keep your tone positive and upbeat (even if your child's isn't). Resign yourself to the idea that, at least for a few weeks, you cannot accomplish anything else during mandatory homework each day. Don't expect fast progress. Think of this as an investment of your time and effort that will pay off in the long run. Also see Chapter 17 for how to remain calm when interacting with a stressful child. In addition, be sure to explain the rationale for mandating homework to your child. Help him or her understand that you are just trying to instill good school-related habits to increase success at school.

Strategy 2: Teaching Your Child Time Management

Infuse time management methods into mandatory homework time. For example, creating a homework checklist at the beginning of each mandatory homework session gives your child a tool to guide work that day and further practice time management. This checklist should contain tasks pertaining to getting things done that are due soon, organizing and planning for the future, and reviewing what was learned in the past. On this checklist your child should write down and then check off:

- What needs to be done for tomorrow

- What needs to be organized, such as school materials, backpack, notebook folders, etc.

- Tasks that require planning, such as longer-term assignments, studying for upcoming tests

- What needs to be reviewed

This is also a good time for writing tasks and due dates into a calendar and/or planner. It can also be productive to check school websites for assignments and tests and then plan accordingly.

Now ask your child to estimate how much time should be devoted to each task on the checklist. For example, an elementary-age child could assign 15 minutes for a math worksheet due tomorrow, 10 minutes for organizing a backpack and folders, 5 minutes for rehearsing spelling words, etc. A teen could assign 30 minutes to work on a term paper outline, 20 minutes for a geography worksheet, 10 minutes to update a planner and organize papers, 20 minutes to review for a social studies test, etc. Then it is up to the child to complete the tasks on the homework checklist and hopefully within the allocated time intervals.

It can also be useful to develop broader time management skills, especially in overly busy older children and teens! Successful students at this age are able to juggle many activities and find sufficient time for school-related tasks. One strategy to assist in managing all of these activities is to create a weekly schedule and follow it to make sure everything gets done. You could create a **standard weekly schedule** that denotes days of the week across the top row and time of day down the far left column. The grid in the middle can then be used to schedule activities, including wake-up time, after-school activities, job, homework, chores, exercise, relaxation (fun activities, down time, favorite TV show, etc.), community activities, worshipping, family time, bedtime, etc. You could also use a **flexible weekly schedule,** on which you plan and write down activities on a week-to-week basis on a calendar or planner.

 TROUBLESHOOTING TIP
Unexpected things come up all the time. Therefore it's always wise to be flexible in the use of schedules. Use them as general guidelines, but be open to changing them as situations develop.

Using calendars and/or planners (paper or electronic) to keep track of the due dates of assignments is also a good idea. Teach your child during mandatory homework time to keep track of his or her assignments and due dates on a daily basis. Each day, ask your child to look at what is due the next day, and look ahead to see what is due in the future, and plan accordingly.

TROUBLESHOOTING TIP
Some children have no idea about due dates for assignments and projects. Nonetheless each day during mandatory homework time you should review all of your child's subjects and ask him or her to take a best guess about tasks and due dates. This will at least get your child oriented to the task of planning. If you keep this up, your child will gradually get better at planning accurately.

Strategy 3: Teaching Your Child Organizational and Planning Skills

Make organizing and planning activities part of mandatory homework activities.

Keeping the Environment Organized

You've heard the saying "A place for everything and everything in its place." There is a lot of wisdom in that idea, especially for a child struggling with academics.

Work with your child to get the home environment and homework area well organized. Make sure that paper, pencils, computer accessories, etc., are all on hand. Use labeled bins to keep track of papers and other school-related materials. Use a bulletin board to pin up lists, assignment directions, miscellaneous papers, and so forth. Hang up a calendar for easy reference. Occasionally clean up and discard papers and other trash to avoid distracting clutter.

Using a Folder System

With assignment directions, worksheets, handouts, reports, and essays, children need to keep track of a lot of school-related paperwork. Many folder systems are available for keeping all of this organized. They usually consist of pockets where paperwork can be collected. With younger children it might be useful to have "To School" and "To Home" pockets, with paperwork filed accordingly. Older children and teens might find it useful to have a folder for each class, with each folder containing "In Progress" and "Needs to Be Turned in" pockets, with paperwork filed accordingly. The folders are best kept in backpacks so that they can be used at school and at home and are readily accessible.

Using Task Checklists

In addition to the daily checklist procedure built into the mandatory homework time procedure, your child (especially an older child or a teen) could stay organized using a **big assignment to-do list.** Essentially the list includes all the smaller tasks necessary to complete a longer-term project. For example, a big assignment to-do list for a class term paper might include:

- Search the Internet for five articles on Thursday, February 26.

- Read and take notes on the five articles on Sunday, March 1.

- Create an outline for the paper on Monday, March 2.

- Write a draft on Tuesday and Wednesday, March 3–4.

- Edit and finalize the paper on Thursday, March 5.

- Hand in paper on Friday, March 6.

These could also be noted on a calendar or planner (see Strategy 2).

Using Reminder Notes

Little notes strategically placed can help your child remember things. Place reminder sticky notes on the edge of a computer screen or on a bulletin board. Place a reminder note on the kitchen table at night so that your child will see it in the morning. Put a note in your child's backpack to remind him or her of things to do at school, such as hand in assignments or ask the teacher a question. Sometimes you may need to do all of the above!

Strategy 4: Teaching Your Child Reviewing Skills

Incorporate reviewing activities into each mandatory homework episode.

Many children make careless mistakes on their schoolwork. Mistakes can be minimized by getting the child in the habit of checking work for accuracy. Designate 5 or 10 minutes at the end of mandatory homework time for the child to double-check what was accomplished.

Some children have difficulty remembering things and consolidating what they learn in school. Systematically reviewing information can help. Many children need to visually review spelling words, math problems, readings, lecture notes, and other material. For an older child or teen, reviewing each academic subject periodically to keep up on what is being taught is also a good habit to cultivate. Help your child develop a routine of reviewing a different subject each day for 5 or 10 minutes. For example, the child could review math facts one night, social studies another night, etc.

Flash cards are very helpful for memorizing and in preparing for upcoming tests. Have your child write his or her own questions (based on readings, lecture notes, etc.) on one side of a note card and then the answer on the other side. The child can review the flash cards until the material is mastered. Alternatively, a voice-type "flash card" could be created (instead of a note card) by voice-recording verbally stated questions (based on readings, lecture notes, etc.), pausing for a few moments, and then verbally answering the question. Later the child can listen to the voice recording and answer the questions during the previously recorded pauses.

Strategy 5: Teaching Your Child to Stay On Task

You can teach your child to monitor his or her own on-task behavior during mandatory homework time.

Step 1: Teaching On-Task Behavior

"On task" can be a foreign concept for a child, so be sure that your child understands clearly what being on task entails. For example, with homework, explain that on-task behavior is looking at one's work, having the pencil touch the paper, writing, calculating, or reading. If explanations don't seem to be enough, model the behavior. You can actually sit at a desk or table and physically demonstrate.

Step 2: Using Self-Monitoring for On-Task Behavior

The *Staying On Task* form (at the end of this chapter) can be used to help your child increase on-task behavior.

- Assign a task and time interval for your child to complete it.

- Fill in the *Staying On Task* form with your child.

For example: At the end of homework time, both you and your child rate how well he or she stayed on task according to the 5-point rating on the *Staying On Task* form.

At first it is not so important that your child actually improve at being on task. What's most important early on is that your ratings match. Coming up with the same ratings as you shows that your child is becoming a better observer of his or her own behavior and more aware of being on or off task. You could give your child a reward if the rating matches yours on the *Staying On Task* form.

The next step is to use the *Staying On Task* chart to improve on-task behavior. **Now you want your child to actually obtain ratings of 3, 4, or 5 on the chart.** You could give your child a small reward for achieving a good rating on the *Staying On Task* chart.

Note: *After the child has mastered the **Staying On Task** procedure at home, it can be used at school if the teacher will support it.*

Achieving Success with School Survival Skills

School survival skills involve learning and using strategies to manage time, organize, plan, review, and stay on task in order to do better at school. This chapter provides ideas and strategies for helping your child develop these skills and, in turn, becoming more successful at school. To follow through, periodically review the *Parent Checklist for School Survival Skills* at the end of this chapter or set your own goals to attain with the *Parenting Goals* form at the end of Chapter 3. It is also a good idea to encourage your child to set specific school survival goals ("Fill out my planner every school day," "Practice staying on task during homework," etc.) and monitor progress on the *Personal Goals (Basic* or *Advanced)* form at the end of Chapter 3. Consider providing rewards to your child for trying the new school survival skills (see Chapter 3 for more ideas on motivating your child).

The mandatory homework time is arguably the most important strategy in this chapter because it provides an opportunity not only to get homework done but also to practice other school survival skills. Make sure that you follow through with mandatory homework time for the long haul. You need to be **persistent** and **consistent** (i.e., PERCON) in applying these skills-building strategies every day until they work. Sometimes this takes weeks or months.

Parent Checklist for School Survival Skills

Name: _____ **Date:** _____

In the blanks below, indicate a score for **how well** you make use of that parenting behavior at this time.

Not too well	**Okay**	**Very well**
1	**2**	**3**

Parent's Efforts in Using Mandatory Homework Time with Child

A. ____ Using a mandatory homework time that focuses on getting things done that are due, organizing and planning for future assignments, and reviewing past school material

B. ____ Checking in with the child as homework begins and checking out with the child as homework ends

C. ____ Incorporating some stress management techniques into a mandatory homework session

D. ____ Providing assistance in a calm manner to make sure that things get done during mandatory homework time

Parent's Efforts in Teaching School Survival Skills to Child

E. ____ Teaching time management skills, like writing down tasks and estimating time during homework; and/or using a weekly schedule, calendars, or planners

F. ____ Teaching organization and planning skills, like creating an organized study area at home and/or using a folder system and/or using task checklists and/or using reminder notes

G. ____ Teaching reviewing by facilitating a habit of checking work for accuracy during homework time and developing a routine of reviewing different academic subjects each day

H. ____ Teaching on-task behavior, like self-monitoring, to improve on-task behavior during homework time

Staying On Task

Name: _____ **Date:** _____

Indicate below what task you will be doing (e.g., schoolwork, cleaning up your desk, a special project) and the time period you will be working on the task. After you have completed the task, or after the time period is over, rate yourself as to how well you stayed on task. Next a parent should rate how well you stayed on task.

Task to Be Completed and Time Period

1. I will work on this task during this time:

Child Evaluation

2. How well did I stay on task? (Circle one.)

1	2	3	4	5
Not at all	A little	Okay	Pretty well	Great

Parent Evaluation

3. How well did child stay on task? (Circle one.)

1	2	3	4	5
Not at all	A little	Okay	Pretty well	Great

Reward

4. If my rating matches my parent rating, I get this reward:

OR

5. If my parent rates me as a *3, 4,* or *5,* I get this reward:

16

Teaming Up

Collaborating and Advocating for Your Child at School

Unfortunately, many parents don't find out that their child is struggling at school until they get a call or a note from a teacher. It is frustrating to learn that your child has missing assignments, poor grades, or has been disruptive in the classroom. Parents often feel helpless because they do not know how to help their child at school. You can influence your child's school behavior and academic progress, however, by effectively teaming up with school officials. This chapter provides ideas for some of the best ways to work with schools.

Note: *Although the focus of this chapter is ultimately about the child, it is the parent who will be doing most of the work in teaming up.*

Choosing a Focus for Teaming Up at School

Start by using the *Parent Checklist for Teaming Up at School* (at the end of this chapter) to pinpoint where you are now and focus on what needs work. This checklist will also provide an overview of the topics covered in this chapter. You can refer to the checklist periodically for reminders and to measure your progress.

Strategy 1: Effectively *Collaborating* at School

It is essential to form a team consisting of at least the parent(s) and teacher(s). Other school personnel, such as the school psychologist, counselor, social worker, and principal, might also be team members. Sometimes a child will be on the team if he or she is cooperative. This team can be informal or a formalized "Student Intervention Team" (in some schools, this team has a different name). To help your child succeed at school, this team must collaborate effectively and come up with a plan of specific interventions.

Establishing Communication with the School

Find out the best way to communicate with the teacher(s) and other school personnel. Some of these people are easiest to reach by phone, others by e-mail, and others prefer face-to-face meetings. Once you have reached them, you can ask about your child's academic and behavioral progress. **During conversations, it is helpful to avoid blaming and share your desire to work with school staff to support your son or daughter.**

Identifying Problem Behaviors and Devising a Plan of Action

Define the problem behaviors and determine what can be done. Ask a few questions to figure out exactly what is going on, including:

- What does the behavior look like?
- When does it happen?
- When does it not happen?
- Who else is involved?

- How long has this behavior been going on?
- How have the teacher and school staff responded to the behavior?

Now that you know what the problem behaviors are, the team should brainstorm about specific strategies to alter these behaviors. One strategy is to teach and reinforce alternative or "replacement" behaviors in your child. The following are some common problem behaviors and corresponding replacement behaviors:

Problem Behaviors

- Talking out loud without permission
- Talking with peers during instruction

Replacement Behaviors

- Raising hand and waiting to be called on
- Remaining quiet during instruction unless called upon by the teacher

- Out of seat during instruction

- Sitting in seat during instructional activities until given permission to get up

- Not turning in homework

- Turning in homework within 5 minutes of arriving in class after one reminder from teacher

- Not listening to teacher's instructions

- Looking at teacher and listening to instructions

- Copying peers' work

- Completing work independently with eyes on own paper

- Off-task and disruptive during independent seatwork

- On-task, looking at and completing assigned task, during independent seatwork

- Not completing class work

- Completing assigned work in class and requesting help or extra time if needed

The replacement behaviors can then be recast as behavior goals for a child to work on at school. In many instances it is helpful to teach the behavioral goals by explicitly explaining them and by using demonstrations and role playing. For example, describe and show "listening to instructions" in terms of eye contact, body posture, and asking questions of the teacher.

Creating a System of School–Home Communication

A school–home note system can help in monitoring your child's progress at school. The basic idea is to have a note passed between parent(s) and teacher(s) each day with your child acting as the delivery agent. The note provides your child with immediate feedback from the teacher about how well the goals are being met and gives you an opportunity to influence school behavior. The school–home note should specify:

- Behavior goals that your child will work on at school. It is best to focus on two or three behavior goals at most.

- Time intervals when your child will be evaluated as to whether behavior goals are being met. For a younger child it could be once in the morning and once in the afternoon. For an older child or teen it might be every class period.

- Some system for communicating the child's performance of the desired behaviors (e.g., *poor, fair, good*).

The teacher signs the form at the end of the day and sends it home via the child. At first it may be hard for your child to remember to bring the note home, but over time he or she can learn to deliver school–home notes successfully. You might consider administering a mild consequence to your child if he or she repeatedly forgets the note.

It may be a good idea to make typical privileges at home conditional on school behavior each day (if desired and feasible). For example, a child who has a good day at school (e.g., 80% "fair" or "good" evaluations by teachers) can keep home privileges for the next 24 hours; otherwise the child will lose some of them. Privileges that could be removed include access to video games, computer, television, cell phone, iPod, going out with friends, or the use of the car for an older teen. Privileges lost one day can be earned back the next day with a good teacher evaluation.

Consider providing "bonus rewards" to motivate your child to do well each day in school. For example, your child could earn a token for each really good day (e.g., 80% "good" evaluations by teachers), and these tokens could be "cashed in" for extra rewards such as going to a movie or having a pizza party on the weekend. See Chapter 3 for more reward ideas.

Many teachers already have school–home notes developed, and/or the school psychologist could assist in designing a specific method that is feasible and useful. Two examples—one that could be used or modified for a younger child and the other for an older child or teen—are provided on page 212–214.

Maintaining Ongoing Informal Contact with School Personnel

Whenever possible, try to attend school functions, whether school conferences, day visits, meetings, or activities with which your child is involved during and after school. Most schools have websites that allow teachers to post notes to parents and provide information about homework assignments and grades. Check the website on a regular basis to keep tabs on what is going on in your child's classroom(s). To be truly involved, you should have active and ongoing contact with teacher(s) and school personnel, not just when problems arise.

PRACTICE EXERCISE
It is a good idea to practice what you want to say and how you want to say it before you communicate with a teacher or school official. Write down the main points you wish to get across. Consider actually rehearsing before you communicate.

Strategy 2: Effectively *Advocating* at School

Sometimes it is necessary to access special help at the school. This section gives you information and strategies for being an effective advocate for your child at school.

Getting Help at School

There are many places to go for help at school. It is best to start with your child's teacher. In addition, the school psychologist, principal, or district special education director should be able to provide you with detailed information about the special education referral and evaluation process, eligibility decisions, and an individualized education program (IEP).

Often it is necessary to attend school meetings to get help for your child. These meetings can be intimidating for parents, so it is best to be prepared. When you go to a meeting, it is important to be on time so that you have the maximum amount of time scheduled to discuss problems and solutions. Take along a list of your concerns (e.g., spending too long on homework, never bringing homework home, failing grades) and remedies attempted so far at home. If your child has been evaluated by a medical doctor, psychologist, or other professional who has determined that your child has a condition that might impact school performance, take along copies of reports or other relevant records.

Knowing Your Rights and the Process to Obtain Them

Federal laws, such as the Individuals with Disabilities Education Improvement Act (IDEIA) and Section 504 of the Rehabilitation Act of 1973, require the public education system to provide services for youth who have emotional, behavioral, or learning problems that limit their ability to succeed in school. To receive these services, a child must be referred to a multidisciplinary school team to assess the need for evaluation. If the multidisciplinary team concludes that an evaluation is in order, you will be asked to sign a consent form to begin the process. The evaluation procedure varies from school to school and from child to child. Consenting to an evaluation does not require you to agree with the results or plan. At the end of the evaluation, the multidisciplinary team will schedule a meeting to review its findings and discuss recommendations.

The main goal of the evaluation is to determine whether your child is eligible for specialized school services and to focus the resulting plan. There are many categories of special education eligibility, but youth who struggle with behavioral or emotional functioning and/or learning often fall into one of the following categories:

- **Specific learning disability (SLD).** Eligibility for the SLD category means that a child is functioning significantly below age- or grade-level expectations in the area(s) of understanding or using language, reading, writing, and/or math.

- **Emotional–behavioral disorder (EBD) or emotional disturbance (ED).** The EBD or ED category requires longstanding problems with behavioral and/or emotional functioning that negatively impact learning and/or social interactions at school.

- **Other health impairment (OHI).** To receive services under the OHI category, a child must have a medical diagnosis **and** be struggling in school as a result of this diagnosis. Documentation can come in the form of a diagnosis from your child's pediatrician, psychologist, or psychiatrist.

- **Developmental delay (DD).** The DD category is used for a child who is 3–9 years old and is demonstrating deficits requiring special education or related services in one or more of the following developmental areas: physical, cognitive, communication, social–emotional, and adaptive functioning.

- **Autism spectrum disorder (ASD).** This category represents a developmental disability that significantly impacts verbal and nonverbal communication, social interaction, and school performance. This developmental disability is usually evident before the age of 3.

- **Intellectual disability (ID).** Eligibility for the ID category requires significantly subaverage intellectual and adaptive functioning that negatively impacts school performance.

- **Traumatic brain injury (TBI).** A child is eligible for this category if he or she sustained an external brain injury resulting in total or partial functional disability and/or associated impairment in school performance.

You will be informed whether your child is eligible for one or more of these special education services. This eventually leads to the development of an IEP by you and the multidisciplinary team, which will identify how, where, and how much specially designed instruction your child will receive. You must provide consent before these services begin.

Ask for What Your Child Needs

If your child qualifies for assistance with behavior problems, you can ask that specific techniques be used by school personnel to improve your child's behavior at school. The ***Behavior Improvement Strategies That Might Be Used at School*** chart (at the end of this chapter) provides ideas that might be considered for your child. It can be helpful to share this list of school strategies with behavior specialist staff at the school. The techniques could be part of your child's official school plan, and/or a behavior specialist staff member could consult with a teacher on how to use them.

If your child has a medical or psychological diagnosis, but does not qualify for special education services, you could ask the school to develop a plan in accordance with **Section 504 of the Rehabilitation Act of 1973**. A 504 plan identifies accommodations that your child will be provided to allow equal access to educational opportunities. Section 504 plans are not part of special education, and no special funding is set aside for them; however, accommodations agreed to in a 504 plan are required by law. A nonexhaustive list of accommodation examples that could be considered is provided in the ***Accommodations That Might Be Used at School*** chart (at the end of this chapter). It is also possible for your child to access special education services under IDEIA and accommodations under Section 504 at the same time.

Being a Team Member

Keep working with the team until you come up with a plan that you think is best for your child. Stay in close contact with the teacher(s) and school personnel. Try to have a friendly and cooperative attitude, but also be assertive as needed in advocating for your child at school.

 PRACTICE EXERCISE
It is helpful to practice what you want to say and how you want to say it before you advocate for your child at school. The suggested strategy is to write down what you want to say and then rehearse it before you say it.

Achieving Success with Teaming Up at School

Teaming up at school means that you are working effectively with school officials on your child's behalf. This chapter provides ideas and strategies for communicating and advocating effectively at school. To follow through, periodically review the *Parent Checklist for Teaming Up at School* at the end of this chapter or set your own goals to attain with the *Parenting Goals* form at the end of Chapter 3.

Perhaps the most important take-home message in this chapter is the value of forming good relationships with school officials so you'll be more effective in communicating and advocating for your child. Putting in the extra effort to accomplish this is well worth a parent's time. You need to be **persistent** and **consistent** (i.e., PERCON) in applying these skills-building strategies every day until they work. Sometimes this takes weeks or months.

Parent Checklist for Teaming Up at School

Name: _____ Date: _____

In the blanks below, indicate a score for **how well** you make use of that parenting behavior at this time.

	Not too well	Okay	Very well
	1	2	3

Parent's Efforts in Effectively *Collaborating* at School

A. _____ Finding out the best way to communicate with teacher(s) and other school personnel (phone, e-mail, face-to-face meetings, etc.)

B. _____ Asking school officials to go beyond just talking about the child's problems to defining "target behaviors," teaching/reinforcing "replacement behaviors," and using other behavioral strategies at school

C. _____ Using a school–home note system about the child's school behavior(s)

D. _____ Maintaining ongoing contact with teacher(s) and school personnel, not just when problems arise

Parent's Efforts in Effectively *Advocating* at School

E. _____ Actively working with school officials to develop and implement a plan for the child's success at school

F. _____ Becoming familiar with federal laws and related procedures to get the public education system to provide services for the child

G. _____ Staying in close contact with teacher(s) and school personnel while trying to have a friendly and cooperative attitude

H. _____ Being assertive (not aggressive) as needed in advocating for the child at school

School–Home Note for a Child

Name: _____ Date: _____

Morning

Behavior Goals   **Circle one**

                                     ☹   😐   🙂

_____   Poor   Fair   Good

_____   Poor   Fair   Good

_____   Poor   Fair   Good

Comments: _____

Teacher's signature: _____

Afternoon

Behavior Goals   **Circle one**

                                     ☹   😐   🙂

_____   Poor   Fair   Good

_____   Poor   Fair   Good

_____   Poor   Fair   Good

Comments: _____

Teacher's signature: _____

Today's homework assignments are:

_____

_____

_____

School–Home Note for an Older Child or Teen

Name: _____ Date: _____

First Class

Behavior Goals	Circle one		
_____	Poor	Fair	Good
_____	Poor	Fair	Good
_____	Poor	Fair	Good

Comments: _____

Teacher's signature: _____

Second Class

Behavior Goals	Circle one		
_____	Poor	Fair	Good
_____	Poor	Fair	Good
_____	Poor	Fair	Good

Comments: _____

Teacher's signature: _____

Third Class

Behavior Goals	Circle one		
_____	Poor	Fair	Good
_____	Poor	Fair	Good
_____	Poor	Fair	Good

Comments: _____

Teacher's signature: _____

(cont.)

Fourth Class

Behavior Goals	**Circle one**		
_____	Poor	Fair	Good
_____	Poor	Fair	Good
_____	Poor	Fair	Good

Comments: _____

Teacher's signature: _____

Fifth Class

Behavior Goals	**Circle one**		
_____	Poor	Fair	Good
_____	Poor	Fair	Good
_____	Poor	Fair	Good

Comments: _____

Teacher's signature: _____

Sixth Class

Behavior Goals	**Circle one**		
_____	Poor	Fair	Good
_____	Poor	Fair	Good
_____	Poor	Fair	Good

Comments: _____

Teacher's signature: _____

Behavior Improvement Strategies That Might Be Used at School

Relationship Building and Catching 'Em Being Good: Disciplining a student is much more effective if the adult has a good relationship with him or her. Avoid critical comments and a frustrated voice tone when talking to the student. Make an extra effort to establish rapport with the child and be sure to praise positive behavior. Strive to make three or more positive comments for every one correction or reprimand.

Behavioral Contracting: Clearly specify behavioral expectations and rewards/consequences associated with meeting behavioral expectations. Devise a behavior progress form with behavioral goals stated, a method for evaluating progress (e.g., one to five ratings), and contingent rewards/consequences for indicated behaviors. It is best to get student input into the selection of reinforcers.

Check-In/Check-Out with Adult Mentor at School: Define behavioral goals with the student and teacher(s) and designate them on a goal chart. Mentor monitors behavioral progress at school. Mentor checks in with student for 5–30 minutes at the beginning of day and checks out with the student for 5–30 minutes at end of day regarding progress with behavioral goals. Mentor forms a positive relationship with the student and uses their relationship to give feedback and engage the student in problem solving about reaching behavioral goals.

Individualized "School Survival Skills" Training:

- *Time Management Skills:* Provide instruction on time budgeting with tasks and creating and following a daily or weekly schedule. Encourage/reward the student for using the skills.

- *Organizational and Planning Skills:* Provide instruction on using calendars to keep track of dates, using task checklists to monitor task completion, and using a folder system to organize schoolwork. Encourage and reward the student for using the skills.

- *Staying On-Task:* Define task-specific indicators of on-task behavior and provide instruction on self-monitoring of on-task behavior. Encourage and reward the student for using the skills.

Management of Noncompliant Behavior: When compliance is needed, give an *effective command* (clear, specific, one-step with eye contact and voice tone raised slightly). If there is no compliance with an effective command, then give a *warning* in the form of an "if . . . then" statement ("if you don't [command], then [time-out chair or time-out room or loss of small privilege]"). If there is no compliance after the warning, *follow through* with what was stated in the warning. Avoid power struggles and deescalate if needed. This procedure works best if the adult doing it has a good relationship and rapport with the student.

Management of Angry Outbursts:

- *Proactive Maintenance of Calm in Student.* Have predictable classroom routines and clearly stated rules and expectations.

- *Proactive Redirecting with Increasing Agitation in Student.* Use calming strategies such as guiding use of stress management, allowing the student to go to "cool down" area.

- *Reactive Management of Outbursts in the Student.* Isolate and remove others from the angry/acting-out student and get help. After calming down, the student should restore the environment and/or make restitution.

Deescalate to Avoid Power Struggles: When the student is agitated, stay calm, minimize verbal commands and directives, reduce eye contact, turn away, and walk away. Do not add consequences. Once calm, reengage the student regarding behavior expectations.

Note: *An educational and/or behavior specialist may need to be involved in implementing these strategies at school.*

From *Skills Training for Struggling Kids.* Copyright 2013 by The Guilford Press.

Accommodations That Might Be Used at School

- Place the student in a low-distraction location in the classroom.

- Use multimodal instruction by presenting information in a variety of ways (auditory, visual, and tactile)

- Fully explain what will be graded for each assignment and what should be focused on before starting an assignment (e.g., spelling, creativity, neatness, showing work).

- Provide instructions for assignments orally and in writing.

- Provide prompt and frequent positive reinforcement for desired behaviors, including beginning tasks, staying on task, and completing assignments.

- Give corrective statements in a brief, immediate, calm, and matter-of-fact tone of voice.

- Provide opportunities to move around the classroom.

- Structure class time to include frequent breaks contingent upon reaching short-term goals.

- Allow extra time to complete tasks and exams/tests in the classroom.

- Shorten some assignments.

- Allow time and provide assistance for the child to do homework at school.

Enhancing Your Well-Being as a Parent

17

You Parent the Way You Think
Thinking Helpful Thoughts to Enhance Parenting

The way you think about your child, your family, and yourself shapes how you respond in parenting situations. For example, if you think, "My child is the cause of our family's problems," you might engage in parenting differently from a parent who thinks "We all have a role in causing our family's problems." The first thought might be unhelpful because it can lead to blaming the child, whereas the second thought might be more helpful because it can lead to a shared sense of responsibility. **Whether or not the thoughts are true is less important than whether or not the thoughts are helpful!** A child may indeed cause many family problems, but that point of view may not help in solving those problems. This chapter will give you ideas for how to examine your thinking in order to have more helpful parent thoughts.

Choosing a Focus for Helpful Parent Thoughts

Start by using the *Parent Checklist for Helpful Parent Thoughts* (at the end of this chapter) to pinpoint where you are now and focus on what needs work. This checklist will also provide an overview of what the topics covered in this chapter are about. You can refer to the checklist periodically for reminders and to measure your progress.

Strategy 1: Promoting Awareness of Your Thinking as a Parent

Let's begin by identifying and examining some unhelpful parent thoughts and consider how they might affect parenting. The *Unhelpful Parent Thoughts* form (at the end of this chapter) can be used to help you understand the effects of unhelpful thoughts on parenting. **The key issue here is not whether the thoughts are accurate (your child may indeed behave like a brat sometimes) but whether the thoughts are helpful.** The thoughts on the *Unhelpful Parent Thoughts* form often result in negative feelings and unproductive parenting behaviors.

Now consider some potentially helpful parent thoughts. The *Helpful Parent Thoughts* (at the end of this chapter) can be used to help you understand the effects of helpful thoughts on parenting. The thoughts on the *Helpful Parent Thoughts* chart often result in positive feelings and productive parenting behaviors.

The basic point is to understand that the way you think can influence your parenting in a positive or negative direction. **Now ask yourself if you tend to have unhelpful or helpful thoughts when it comes to parenting.** It may be a good idea to learn helpful parent thinking skills.

Strategy 2: Working on Your Helpful Parent Thinking

Sometimes parents get in the habit of having mostly unhelpful parent thoughts. If you are such a parent, and you want to change your way of thinking, it may be a good idea to make a conscious effort to do so in your day-to-day family life.

The *Helpful Thoughts Worksheet for Parents* (at the end of this chapter) can be used to guide you through helpful parent thinking steps. When a challenging parenting event occurs (e.g., your child defies a direct command to do the dishes), ask yourself all of the questions on the worksheet to examine and change any unhelpful thoughts.

Try to use the worksheet every day for a week or two so that helpful parent thinking can become a habit.

 PRACTICE EXERCISE
It can be helpful to role-play different scenarios and then practice helpful parent thinking. Perhaps get another adult to act as your child or just practice while looking in the mirror. You can fill out the Helpful Thoughts Worksheet for Parents while you practice. For example, you've asked your child to turn off the TV and come to dinner, but there is no movement! The first thought that pops into your mind is "I'm sick and tired of that brat!" Then you pause and go through the helpful thoughts sequence:

> *1. Am I thinking unhelpful parent thoughts, and if so, what are they? "Yes, I'm thinking that I can't take it because he [she] acts like a brat so much."*

2. *How do my unhelpful parent thoughts make me feel about and act toward my child and family? "I feel angry and will soon be yelling and criticizing him [her] if I don't change this way of thinking."*

3. *Why is it unhelpful to keep thinking this parent thought? "It makes me overreact and leads to a lot of conflicts between us."*

4. *What are different or more helpful parent thoughts I can think? "I need to remain calm and handle this in a firm yet positive manner. I'll give him [her] a warning to turn off the TV and come to dinner or else lose TV for the rest of the evening."*

5. *How do my helpful parent thoughts make me feel about, and act toward, my child and family? "I'm less angry and more effective in handling the situation."*

6. *Why is it helpful to keep thinking this new parent thought? "It will cut down on the negative interactions I have with him [her]."*

 TROUBLESHOOTING TIP
The most common problem with keeping your parenting thoughts helpful is that when you get upset or frustrated, you tend to forget all about helpful thinking. Research and experience inform us that we do not think straight when angry, nervous, agitated, etc. It is imperative to calm down in order to think in a helpful way. With this in mind, make an effort to stay calm when interacting with your child so that you can think straight and have an accurate perspective. Remember to "chill before thinking" so you can respond to parent challenges in the best way possible. See Chapter 18 for more ideas on managing stress and staying calm.

AVOIDING HOPELESSNESS

Feeling defeated and hopeless at times is understandable. After all, the problems can appear endless, and sometimes it seems that what you have tried so far has not helped. But dwelling on how bad things are is counterproductive and leads only to a continuation or worsening of the problems. It can also set a negative tone for parent–child interactions and within the family unit as a whole. No matter how hard it is, you have to have a "can-do" attitude and keep on trying! Focus on accomplishing one or two realistic goals at a time.

FOCUSING PARENT WORRIES WITH THE FUNNEL TECHNIQUE

Too Many Worries and No Focus

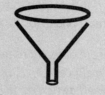

Focus on Something

At times parents worry so much that they become stuck—not knowing what to do next—and this can lead to further inaction. The Funnel Technique involves funneling all of those worries down into one or two focus areas at a time. Don't dwell on everything; focus on one or two important concerns and set about coming up with a plan and putting it into action.

Strategy 3: Working on Your Middle Path Parent Thinking

Parenting a struggling child often entails making changes and taking action. This can be productive and useful as long as it is put into proper perspective. Along with making changes, it can help to accept things as they are and live in the moment. In other words, it is possible to work on changes while striking a balance of acknowledging where you and your family are and being tuned in to what you have each day. This is a state of mind you can adopt as a form of helpful thoughts.

The basic idea is to develop a "middle path" view of seeking change while also fostering acceptance of your child and yourself at the same time. In this way you are going down a middle path of trying to change things but also recognizing and accepting your limitations. Here are some examples of *middle path parenting thoughts*:

- "I can change only so much, and the rest I have to accept."

- "I'll keep plugging away, but I also have to be patient because it takes time to make changes."

- "As long as my child and I are moving in the right direction, it is okay."

- "Some things I can change, and some things I have to accept as they are."

- "I have to look for and notice the small improvements we have made."

- "We have a way to go, but we are seeing some growth."

- "I'm doing the best I can, and there is only so much I can do."

This middle path is a particularly useful point of view considering how child development unfolds slowly over time and how slowly change can sometimes occur. Helpful middle path parenting thoughts can relieve some pressure and keep you calm when you are with your child.

Achieving Success with Helpful Parent Thoughts

Helpful thinking in parents involves recognizing unhelpful thoughts and changing them to make them more helpful. This chapter provides strategies for thinking helpful thoughts. To follow through, periodically review the *Parent Checklist for Helpful Parent Thoughts* at the end of this chapter or set your own goals to attain with the *Parenting Goals* form at the end of Chapter 3. Sometimes it is useful for the parent and child to work on helpful thoughts at the same time using a team approach. You need to be **persistent** and **consistent** (i.e., PERCON) in applying these skills-building strategies every day until they work. Sometimes this takes weeks or months.

Parent Checklist for Helpful Parent Thoughts

Name: _____ Date: _____

In the blanks below, indicate a score for **how well** you make use of that parenting behavior at this time.

Not too well	Okay	Very well
1	2	3

Parent's Efforts in Fostering Helpful Parent Thinking Skills

A. _____ Having awareness of parenting-related thoughts

B. _____ Making a conscious effort to change unhelpful parent thoughts to helpful parent thoughts in day-to-day family life

C. _____ Staying calm while interacting with the child to promote more helpful thinking

Parent's Efforts in Fostering Own Middle Path Parent Thinking

D. _____ Striking a balance between seeking change and fostering acceptance of child and self

Unhelpful Parent Thoughts

Listed below are common thoughts that parents of children with behavioral–emotional problems may have. Read each thought and indicate how frequently that thought (or a similar one) typically occurs for you over an average week. There are no right or wrong answers to these questions. Use the 3-point rating scale to help you answer these questions.

1	2	3
Rarely	Sometimes	Often

Unhelpful Thoughts about My Child

1. ____ My child is behaving like a brat.

2. ____ My child acts up on purpose.

3. ____ My child is the cause of most of our family problems.

4 ____ My child's future is bleak.

5. ____ My child should behave like other children. I shouldn't have to make allowances for my child.

Unhelpful Thoughts about Self/Others

6. ____ It is my fault that my child has a problem.

7. ____ It is his/her fault (other parent) that my child is this way.

8. ____ I can't make mistakes in parenting my child.

9. ____ I give up. There is nothing more I can do for my child.

10. ____ I have no control over my child. I have tried everything.

Unhelpful Thoughts about Who Needs to Change

11. ____ My child is the one who needs to change. All of us would be better off if my child would change.

12. ____ I am the one who needs to change. My family would be better off if I would change.

13. ____ My spouse/partner needs to change. We would all be better off if he/she would change.

14. ____ The teacher needs to change. We would be better off if he/she would change.

15. ____ Medications are the answer. Medications will change my child.

For each thought you rated a *3*, ask yourself the following questions:

1. How does this unhelpful thought make me **feel** about my child and family?

2. How does this unhelpful thought make me **act toward** my child and family?

3. Is this an unhelpful thought that I should be more aware of and try to change?

Helpful Parent Thoughts

Listed below are counterthoughts that parents can think instead of unhelpful thoughts. Unhelpful Thought #1 corresponds to Helpful Thought #1, and so on. Compare the unhelpful thoughts to the helpful thoughts.

Helpful Thoughts about My Child

1. My child is behaving positively too.

2. It doesn't matter whose fault it is. What matters are solutions to the problems.

3. It is not just my child. I also play a role in the problem.

4. I have no proof that my child will continue to have problems. I need to wait for the future.

5. I can't just expect my child to behave. My child needs to be taught how to behave.

Helpful Thoughts about Self/Others

6. It doesn't help to blame myself. I will focus on solutions to the problem.

7. It doesn't matter whose fault it is. I will focus on solutions to the problems.

8. My child is perhaps more challenging to parent than others, and therefore I will make mistakes. I need to accept the fact that I am going to make mistakes.

9. I have to parent my child. I have no choice. I need to think of new ways to parent my child.

10. My belief that I have no control over my child might be contributing to the problem. Many things are in my control. I need to figure out what I can do to parent my child.

Unhelpful Thoughts about Who Needs to Change

11. It's unhelpful to think of my child as the only one needing to change. We all need to change.

12. It's unhelpful to think of myself as needing to change. We all need to change.

13. It's unhelpful to think of my spouse/partner as being the only one who needs to change. We all need to change.

14. It's unhelpful to think that only the teacher needs to change. We all need to work together.

15. Medications may help but will not solve the problems. We will also need to work hard to cope with the problems.

Ask yourself the following questions about each of these helpful thoughts:

1. How does this helpful thought make me **feel** about my child and family?

2. How does this helpful thought make me **act toward** my child and family?

3. Is this a helpful thought that I should be more aware of and try to keep?

Helpful Thoughts Worksheet for Parents

Name: _____ **Date:** _____

Fill out the worksheet during or after you have experienced unhelpful parent thoughts.

1. Am I thinking unhelpful parent thoughts, and if so, what are they?

2. How do my unhelpful parent thoughts make me feel about and act toward my child and family?

3. Why is it unhelpful to keep thinking this parent thought?

4. What are different or more helpful parent thoughts I can think?

5. How do my helpful parent thoughts make me feel about, and act toward, my child and family?

6. Why is it helpful to keep thinking this new parent thought?

How Well Did It Work?

(Circle *1, 2, 3,* or *4.*)

1. **I didn't really try too hard.**
2. **I sort of tried, but it didn't really work.**
3. **I tried hard, and it kind of worked.**
4. **I tried really hard, and it really worked.**

18

Cool Parents

Managing Your Own Stress to Enhance Parenting

It's no secret. We all know that parents who are stressed out have a harder time with parenting! Parent stress is experienced in four primary ways:

- **Personal stress**—you feel overwhelmed by everyday life.

- **Marital/relationship stress**—you and your partner (if applicable) have too much conflict.

- **Parenting stress**—the numerous day-to-day challenges of raising children are getting to you.

- **Little or no social support**—you feel alone and/or get little help with parenting.

The *Parent Stress Cycle* shows how parent stress, parent thoughts (see Chapter 17), parenting, and child struggles are all related. It can become a vicious cycle that is hard to stop.

The take-home message here is that reducing stress can make anyone a better parent! This chapter suggests many ways in which you might manage stress. In so doing you will have more helpful parent thoughts and be more effective in parenting, which in turn should improve your child's overall adjustment, and then lessen your stress.

Choosing a Focus for Parent Stress Management

Start by using the *Parent Checklist for Parent Stress Management* (at the end of this chapter) to pinpoint where you are now and focus on what needs work. This

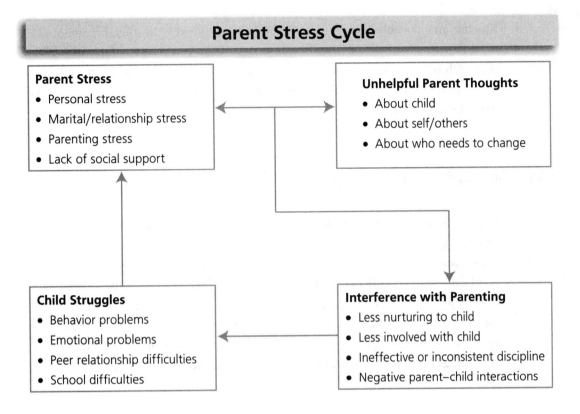

Parent Stress Cycle

Parent Stress
- Personal stress
- Marital/relationship stress
- Parenting stress
- Lack of social support

Unhelpful Parent Thoughts
- About child
- About self/others
- About who needs to change

Child Struggles
- Behavior problems
- Emotional problems
- Peer relationship difficulties
- School difficulties

Interference with Parenting
- Less nurturing to child
- Less involved with child
- Ineffective or inconsistent discipline
- Negative parent–child interactions

checklist will also provide an overview of the topics covered in this chapter. You can refer to the checklist periodically for reminders and to measure your progress.

Strategy 1: Making Stress-Reducing Lifestyle Changes

This strategy is about managing day-to-day stress through regular routines and habits. It involves incorporating healthy behaviors into everyday activities. These commonsense actions are **proactive** ways for keeping one's general stress at a manageable level.

Taking Time Away from Family Responsibility

You may feel like you don't have a moment to spare, or maybe you've just gotten out of the habit of pursuing your own interests. But it can be rejuvenating to schedule time for an enjoyable activity or interest. You may need to arrange for a babysitter, or, if there are two parents, you might want to take turns caring for your child so that each of you can get out occasionally. If this feels impossible, start with really short breaks—like 30 minutes to read a novel or a magazine focused on a hobby you haven't pursued in a while.

Taking Time to Be with Your Spouse/Partner

When you have a child with longstanding behavioral–emotional problems, the first thing to get sacrificed is often your relationship with your spouse or partner (if you have one). Spending whatever time you have together discussing your child can lead to conflict between you and also rob you of the renewal you can get from enjoying each other's company. Making a commitment to spend some time together away from family problems does not have to cost money and may be as simple as a walk or drive together. Talk with your spouse or partner about enjoyable things to do together and schedule time to do them, even if you have to start small.

Spending Special Time with Your Child

Parents these days are often so busy they find it hard to make time for their child outside of working on the child's problems. Make an extra effort to spend time alone with your child to build a quality relationship. You will have fewer problems getting along if you schedule occasional special time devoted to your child, in which he or she chooses a favorite activity to pursue with you (see Chapter 19 for more ideas).

Seeking Out Social Support

Parents who are feeling overwhelmed and isolated can benefit from seeking out active support from family members, neighbors, or mental health professionals. This support could involve talking and sharing feelings with friends or family members, asking for help from friends or family members, joining a parent support group, or even participating in individual or group therapy.

Scheduling Pleasant Events

Stress can be relieved by scheduling pleasant events. For example:

- Attend a concert.

- Go out to dinner with a friend.

- Take the dog for a walk with your child.

- Attend a baseball game with your son or daughter.

- Make time for your favorite hobby or interest.

Developing Good Health Habits

It is universally accepted that increasing one's exercise level, eating a healthy diet, getting enough sleep, and relaxing periodically can improve one's ability to cope with stress. There is also considerable evidence that meditation and yoga have powerful health effects. Investing time in those activities is worthy of serious consideration. Consult professional publications and/or a physician regarding a health promotion program for you.

Joining a Parent Support Group

Many parent groups focus on skills training but also allow parents to share stories and obtain support from each other. Many parents benefit from the support and opportunity to share experiences with other parents who are wrestling with the same issues. If your child has behavioral–emotional problems, you may benefit from joining a parent support group. Consult with a local mental health professional or social service agency about such groups in your community.

 TROUBLESHOOTING TIP
Many parents lead hectic lives and find it hard to make time for stress management. This time crunch problem can be lessened by planning ahead. It may be helpful to sit down once a week (like Sunday evening) and schedule stress management activities for the coming week. For example:

- *Schedule times for going out on "dates" with each other (if you have a spouse or partner).*

- *Plan to visit a sister or cousin or someone else whose company you enjoy and/or who offers support on a consistent weekday evening.*

- *Block out certain weekday mornings or evenings for exercise.*

- *Think about ways to get more involved with your child, such as helping with homework, planning a family outing, attending school events or conferences, or volunteering to help with church or school activities during the coming week.*

By planning you increase the odds of following through with stress-reducing actions!

Strategy 2: Being a Mindful Parent

Mindful parenting focuses your thoughts and attention on being fully present with your child in the moment. It is not technically a relaxation technique, but if you increase mindfulness, the result will be a calmer you and you will end up less stressed.

During mindful parenting moments you let go of preoccupations about what's wrong and/or what needs to be done. Instead you focus only on what is happening right then and there with you and your child. You observe it, without judging it, whether it is good or bad. Some techniques for mindful parenting include:

- *Calming* **down so you can be present.** Take some deep breaths, count to 10, stretch, or walk around a little so you can be calm enough to be in the moment with your child.

- *Accepting* **yourself and your child.** Acknowledge that you and your child have good and bad points and it is what it is. Have compassion for how hard it can sometimes be for both of you.

- *Listening* **to your child.** Pay attention to what your child is saying without thinking of what you want to say. You don't have to agree, but you can really listen to your child's point of view.

- *Attending* **to what is occurring.** Pay attention to what your child and you are doing and saying, how your body feels, what emotions are present, and the sights, sounds, and smells of your immediate surroundings.

To accomplish mindfulness in tense parent–child moments, it is a good idea to **calm down first** (see Strategy 3 below for more suggestions). Tell yourself that you need to "chill out," and then, once calmer, try to remember to tell yourself to be mindful as you interact with your child.

 PRACTICE EXERCISE
Try to be mindful in typical parenting situations. You can be mindful while eating meals, driving in the car, doing a homework project, going for a walk together, and even during times when your child is angry, shouting, etc. During these activities, try not to think or worry. Just focus on being fully present, in that parenting moment, drawing on the four techniques above (calming, accepting, listening, attending).

Strategy 3: Staying Calm When Your Child Stresses You Out

This strategy is very important for managing parenting stress spikes that come up now and then. It involves taking control of stress reactions in the moment. Although these are **reactive** ways for reducing stress, they require a lot of proactive planning and practicing to make them effective under fire.

Step 1: Being Aware of When Your Child Is Stressing You Out

Try to be more aware of your body, thoughts, and actions while interacting with your child. For example, imagine you are getting ready to go to a dentist appointment and you need to get out of the house soon, but your child is very slow to get ready.

- **Body:** You might feel tense, your heart rate speeds up, and you breathe rapidly.

- **Thoughts:** Your thoughts might be unhelpful, such as, "That brat!" "Why do we have to go through the same old stuff every day?" "I'm going to ground him for a year this time!"

- **Action:** In this scenario it would not be too surprising if, out of frustration, you ended up yelling and threatening your child.

Make a list of typical stressful events that occur regularly with your child and what is typical of your body, thought, and action responses.

Step 2: Controlling Your Reactions

The **_Parent Staying Calm_** chart (at the end of this chapter) displays body, thought, and action "signals" that you need to be aware of when dealing with a stressful child.

Staying calm involves learning to control your body, thoughts, and actions in the face of parenting stress. This means learning to:

- Relax your body.

- Think coping thoughts.

- Use imagery.

- Take effective action.

The **_Parent Staying Calm_** chart summarizes ways you can control your body, thoughts, and actions when dealing with stressful situations involving your child. You could post this chart in your house to remind you of what to do.

PRACTICE EXERCISE
*It can be helpful to practice staying calm in different scenarios. Maybe another adult could act as your child. An example of a scenario to use could be when your child is procrastinating with homework. You know it's getting late, and you may need to help out. It is making you irate that your child won't get down to business and get the work done! Now refer to the **Parent Staying Calm** chart. Note the signals that you might experience if you were stressed and tense. Relax your body (e.g., take deep breaths, count to 10), think coping thoughts (e.g., "Okay, I will stay calm and give a warning to get to work or lose TV for 24 hours"), and take effective action (e.g., give the warning and follow through if necessary).*

TROUBLESHOOTING TIP
*A stressed-out child can surely stress out a parent. If your child could just manage his or her own stress, yours would go down (at least to an extent). You can help your child manage stress by learning the strategies outlined in Chapter 14. In addition, you can help your child by modeling good stress management. Whenever you get stressed out, get out the **Parent Staying Calm** chart and go through the steps. It's a good idea to let your child know that you are working on staying calm, so allow your child to see you referring to the **Parent Staying Calm** chart.*

Achieving Success with Parent Stress Management

Parent stress management involves going through steps to cope better with stress that can affect parenting. This chapter provides strategies to use to become a coping parent. To follow through, periodically review the *Parent Checklist for Parent Stress Management* at the end of this chapter or set your own goals to attain with the *Parenting Goals* form at the end of Chapter 3.

Sometimes it is useful for parent and child to work on stress management at the same time using a team approach. You need to be **persistent** and **consistent** (i.e., PERCON) in applying these skills-building strategies every day until they work. Sometimes this takes weeks or months.

Parent Checklist for Parent Stress Management

Name: _____ Date: _____

In the blanks below, indicate a score for **how well** you make use of that parenting behavior at this time.

Not too well	Okay	Very well
1	2	3

Parent's Efforts in Making Stress-Reducing Lifestyle Changes

A. _____ Taking time away from family responsibility

B. _____ Taking time to be with spouse/partner (if applicable)

C. _____ Taking time to be with your child

D. _____ Seeking out social support from friends and/or family

E. _____ Scheduling pleasant events and enjoyable activities

F. _____ Developing good health habits

G. _____ Joining a parent support group

Parent's Efforts in Mindful Parenting

H. _____ Mindfully focusing attention on being fully present with the child in "good" moments

I. _____ Mindfully focusing attention on being fully present with the child in "bad" moments

Parent's Efforts in Staying Calm with the Child

J. _____ Being attentive to body, thought, and behavior signals of stress

K. _____ Controlling your reactions and staying calm by relaxing your body, thinking coping thoughts, using imagery, taking effective action, etc.

Parent Staying Calm

1. **Recognizing Stress**—Be aware of stress "signals."

   Body Signals:

   - Breathing/heart rate increases
   - Tense muscles
   - Increased sweating
   - Face turns red
   - Body feels hot

   Thought Signals:

   - "That brat! I'm not going to take any more!"
   - "I'm a worthless parent."
   - "I give up."
   - "I can't handle this!"
   - "I hate him/her."

   Behavior Signals:

   - Yell/threaten
   - Cry
   - Tremble
   - Withdraw

2. **Relaxing Your Body**—Do deep breathing, tense and release muscles, count to 10, and so forth.

3. **Using "Coping Self-Talk"**—Examples of coping self-talk include the following:

   - "Take it easy."
   - "Don't let it bug you."
   - "I can handle this."
   - "I'm going to be okay."
   - "Stay cool."
   - "Relax."
   - "I'll try my best."

4. **Using Imagery**—Imagine yourself as a robot when your child is stressing you out. Robots execute behavior but have no feelings. Like a robot, execute the behavior of parenting your child while staying cool.

5. **Taking Effective Action**—Walk away, ignore it, take a walk, try to discuss it, express feelings, think of new ways to solve the problem.

Enhancing Your Family's Well-Being

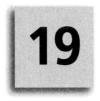

19

Let's Get Together

Strengthening Family Bonds and Organization

Experts agree that families with members who are strongly bonded to each other are more likely to have a successful child. In addition, many children benefit from an organized day-to-day family routine. This chapter will give you ideas for strengthening parent–child bonds through activities, enhancing family connections via rituals, and improving family organization through routines. These are commonsense ideas that do not take too much time yet can be very powerful. Review them all and then select a few for your family.

Choosing a Focus for Family Bonding and Organization

Start by using the *Parent Checklist for Family Bonding and Organization* (at the end of this chapter) to pinpoint where you are now and focus on what needs work. This checklist will also provide an overview of the topics covered in this chapter. You can refer to the checklist periodically for reminders and to measure your progress.

Strategy 1: Strengthening the Parent–Child Bond through Activities

Sometimes parent and child drift apart or family problems like divorce impact bonding in some way. Fortunately, there are many things you can do to improve the bond with your child if you prioritize it and make an effort. In addition to the enjoyment that comes with good parent–child relationships comes the benefit that discipline goes more easily when the bond is strong. For all of these reasons actively working to build the relationship with your child and maintaining it over time is time well spent.

Making Time for Positive Child-Directed Activities

Regularly scheduled positive activities with your child can enhance the bond between you, and they take only a little bit of time each week. Make these activities child-directed, meaning, your child comes up with ideas and you follow along. For example, a young child might choose to play in the sandbox with trucks, whereas an older child or teen might choose to play catch or make cookies. Try the following four steps:

1. List as many activities as you can that your child enjoys doing with you. They should last about a half-hour. Ask your son or daughter for ideas, like:

   - Build something
   - Play with cars/dolls
   - Go for a walk or ride bikes
   - Play catch or work on golf swing
   - Play one-on-one basketball
   - Go shopping
   - Play a game
   - Talk
   - Bake/cook something

2. Schedule one or more 30-minute "appointments" a week to do one or more of these activities together. It can help to agree on a time and mark it on a calendar. If for some reason you can't keep the appointment, be sure to reschedule it. This helps build trust with your child.

3. During the activity, allow your child to be in charge. Make an effort to make positive comments that describe the activities and praise your child, like:

   - "You are stacking the blocks."
   - "You are throwing the ball."
   - "You look happy!"
   - "It looks like you're thinking."
   - "This is fun."
   - "I like doing this with you."
   - "That looks good."
   - "You did a nice job."
   - "Way to go."
   - "Good idea."
   - "That's great!"
   - "It looks nice."

4. Finally, after the activity has been completed, talk about the time you spent together. Listen to what your child has to say and offer positive feedback.

Try this routine for several weeks to get things going. After that, interacting with your child in this positive way may become automatic.

Making Time for Special Conversations

During special talk times, the goal is to focus completely on your child and strive to understand his or her feelings. Try to get your child to talk about interests, feelings, problems, and successes. It may work to do this at dinner or just before bed.

With busy teens it is especially hard to set aside time to talk. Be alert and take advantage of opportunities for special talk time such as while you're in the car together, during a shopping trip, or when doing chores around the house together.

Getting More Involved

Make an effort to become involved in your child's activities and interests, including:

- Attending teacher conferences
- Watching athletic games
- Attending dance or piano recitals
- Going to band concerts
- Attending any other activity in which your child participates

Occasionally, it is good to schedule longer events together to help build a special relationship, including:

- Dinner out
- Weekend camping trip
- Concert or show
- Volunteering together

Get involved with your child's school and learning, including:

- Volunteering in the classroom
- Helping with homework
- Talking to the teacher
- Attending class events or field trips

Strategy 2: Strengthening Family Bonds through Rituals

Family rituals are repeated and organized activities that have special meaning and create a sense of family. Researchers have determined that families who participate in rituals generally function better than families who do not. Below are several lists of possible family rituals.

Routine Family Rituals

- Eating meals together and talking

- Engaging in family activities such as "game night" or "movie night"

- Having bedtime rituals such as reading books, snuggling, etc.

- Participating in regular everyday activities like going for walks, sitting on the patio, etc.

- Going out for breakfast on Saturdays

Special Family Rituals

- Going on special family outings or vacations

- Celebrating birthdays, wedding anniversaries, family holidays, etc.

- Celebrating cultural and/or religious traditions

- Celebrating successes of family members

Community Rituals

- Visiting family, friends, and/or relatives

- Getting involved in neighborhood, community, and/or religious activities

- Getting involved in organized recreational, sports, arts, educational, scouting, and other activities

- Getting involved in school activities

Family rituals can improve the family bond. Strive to create new family rituals or keep up with existing ones.

Strategy 3: Enhancing Family Organization through Routines

Some children need more order, predictability, and structure in their daily lives than others. For some children, if the family is disorganized, the children are too. If you think your child is one who needs more routines, then this section will give you some ideas to consider.

One way to develop family routines is to tighten up procedures at specific times of the day. It can be useful to use a checklist to organize the entire day or specific tasks within the day. Several examples follow to illustrate common routines. You would have to modify them to fit the unique circumstances of your family.

Daily Schedule for School Days

- Get up at 6:30

- Get dressed and eat breakfast by 7:00

- Catch the bus at 7:15

- Relax from 4:00 to 5:00 after school

- Help out with preparations and then eat dinner about 5:15

- Homework from 6:00 to 7:00 or so

- Get ready for bed about 8:00

- In bed by 8:15

- Lights out by 8:30 (or later for an older child or teen)

Getting Ready for School in the Morning

- Get up at 6:30 A.M.

- Take a shower

- Get dressed

- Eat breakfast

- Brush teeth

- Get backpack

- Go catch bus at 7:15 A.M.

Homework

- Begin at 6:00 P.M.

- Get out all books

- Write down all tasks that need to be done

- Ask for help if needed

- Check my work

- End at 7:00 P.M.

Dinnertime

- Set the dinner table
- Clear dishes to counter
- Scrape dishes into trash
- Unload dishes from dishwasher if there are clean dishes in it

- Load dishwasher with dirty dishes and turn on if full
- Clean pots and pans
- Wipe all counters and table

Bedtime

- Begin at specified time each night
- Take a shower or bath
- Put on pajamas
- Brush teeth

- Read a bedtime story
- Talk about the day
- Hugs and kisses
- Lights out at specified time each night

Predictability can also be enhanced by the expectation that the child will contribute to the family by taking on certain **responsibilities,** including:

- Doing chores like dishes, cleaning room, laundry, cleaning messes, etc.
- Taking care of health, like brushing teeth, showering, washing up, etc.

- Helping with pets, including walking the dog, feeding the cat, etc.
- Assisting with shopping and meal preparation, etc.

Achieving Success with Family Bonding and Organization

Families with members who are strongly bonded to each other and who are organized in day-to-day family life are more likely to have a successful child. This chapter provides strategies for shoring up your family's day-to-day functioning to accomplish those goals. To follow through, periodically review the ***Parent Checklist for Family Bonding and Organization*** at the end of this chapter or set your own goals to attain with the ***Parenting Goals*** form at the end of Chapter 3.

After working at this a while, you'll develop good family habits. You need to be **persistent** and **consistent** (i.e., PERCON) in applying these skills-building strategies every day until they work. Sometimes this takes weeks or months.

Parent Checklist for Family Bonding and Organization

Name: _____ Date: _____

In the blanks below, indicate a score for **how well** you make use of that parenting behavior at this time.

	Not too well	Okay	Very well
	1	2	3

Parent's Efforts in Building Parent–Child Bonds Through Activities

A. ____ Making time for positive child-directed activities

B. ____ Making time for special conversations

C. ____ Getting more involved in activities and at school

D. ____ Other (specify): _____

Parent's Efforts in Strengthening Family Bonds through Rituals

E. ____ Making time for regular family rituals

F. ____ Making time for special family rituals

G. ____ Making time for community rituals

H. ____ Other (specify): _____

Parent's Efforts in Enhancing Family Organization through Routines

I. ____ Getting ready for school in the morning

J. ____ Having regular homework time

K. ____ Having regular dinnertime

L. ____ Having regular bedtime

M. ____ Other (specify): _____

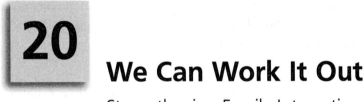

20

We Can Work It Out

Strengthening Family Interaction Skills

Families sometimes fall into bad communication habits and have a hard time solving their everyday problems, and, as a result, conflicts erupt. These interaction difficulties can be destructive to the family unit and have the potential to make family members feel hurt and angry. In contrast, good communication, problem-solving, and conflict resolution skills enable a family to keep operating smoothly. This in turn has a positive effect on the children in the family. This chapter will give you suggestions for improving ongoing family interaction skills.

    Note: Below there are suggestions for conducting family meetings to learn and practice family interaction skills. Such meetings might go better and be more successful with the guidance of a practitioner. Once you have the procedures down, you can have similar meetings at home to review and use the skills.

Choosing a Focus for Family Interactions

Start by using the ***Parent Checklist for Family Interactions*** (at the end of this chapter) to pinpoint where you are now and focus on what needs work. This checklist will also provide an overview of the topics covered in this chapter. You can refer to the checklist periodically for reminders and to measure your progress.

Strategy 1: Working on Family Communication Skills

Step 1: Learning and Practicing Family Communication Skills

Call a family meeting at a time that works for everyone. Explain that the purpose of the meeting is to discuss ways of improving family communication and that no one person is in trouble. Keep it low key. Do not try to solve any big family problems at the meeting. Each family member should be given a copy of the *Family Communication Skills* chart (at the end of this chapter) to review.

- Ask each family member to evaluate him- or herself (**not each other**) to determine which "DON'Ts" each person does too much.

- As long as everyone is still agreeable, ask family members to give one another feedback about specific "DON'Ts" they see each other doing too much.

- Ask family members to identify one or two "DOs" that they will work on to improve family communication.

 PRACTICE EXERCISE

It helps to do a simulated practice of family communication skills. For example, try discussing when homework should be done tonight. **Begin by illustrating ineffective communication so family members can see what that looks like.** *In the spirit of fun, ask family members to pretend and act out the "DON'Ts" on the* **Family Communication Skills** *chart. You may demonstrate a "lecture" by going on and on (e.g., "It is important for you to keep up with homework because when you get older . . . "; "When I was your age . . . ").* **Then use effective communication so members can see what that looks like.** *Ask family members to "act out" the "DOs" on the* **Family Communication Skills** *chart. For example, demonstrate using "brief statements" about homework (e.g., "I expect you to do homework from 5:00 to 6:00 P.M."). As long as everyone is still agreeable, ask each family member to practice "DON'Ts" and "DOs" in this exercise. Family members should strive to coach and support one another as they apply specific skills. Keep practicing until family members feel that they have learned the specified family communication skills.*

Step 2: Using Family Communication Skills at Home

After the family has learned and practiced the family communication skills, try to use them to solve real-life problems. It would be helpful, again, for family members to have the *Family Communication Skills* chart in their hands while carrying on the discussion. Examples of real problems to discuss include issues around homework, house rules, curfew, parents' concerns regarding a child's grades, and child's concerns regarding parents' rules.

Several strategies can be used to help family members use communication skills at home:

- Post copies of the *Family Communication Skills* chart in conveniently accessible places within the home (on refrigerator, bulletin board, etc.).

- Use the *My Family Communication Goals* form (at the end of this chapter). Have family members each identify specific family communication skills goals they will work on and then monitor progress.

- Conduct occasional 10-minute family meetings to review and discuss progress with communication skills.

 PRACTICE EXERCISE
*Try having a family discussion about one of the topics suggested above. Before beginning, ask each family member to set one or two communication goals and designate them on the **My Family Communication Goals** form (at the end of this chapter). Then ask family members to try to work on their goals while discussing the topic. As long as the discussion stays cordial, allow family members to evaluate themselves and critique others regarding how well they each met their goals on the **My Family Communication Goals** form.*

 TROUBLESHOOTING TIP
Occasionally a child will refuse to participate or do so only halfheartedly with family communication skills. Don't fret. You can still change your son or daughter's communication by changing your own. That's because family communication is interactional. For example, your giving a long lecture can result in your child's exhibiting poor listening—and that in turn, makes you prone to sermonize! On the other hand, your use of a brief statement can result in your child's willingness to listen, which in turn reinforces your continued use of brief, to-the-point statements. So keep working at communications skills yourself even if your child is less than cooperative.

Strategy 2: Working on Family Problem-Solving Skills

Step 1: Learning and Practicing Family Problem-Solving Skills

It's time to reconvene another family meeting at a time that is convenient for everyone and where everyone is feeling good about being together. Give everyone a copy of the *Family Problem Solving* chart to look at (at the end of this chapter).

- Ask for opinions about how well everyone thinks the family is able to solve its problems.

- Try to reach a consensus to work on family problem solving.

- Review the family problem-solving steps and make sure that everyone understands them.

After the family problem-solving skills have been introduced, it is a good idea for family members to practice using them to solve neutral or easy problems.

 PRACTICE EXERCISE
At first, try to solve a fun problem such as how to spend an imaginary $1,000,000 that your family just won in the lottery. Next try to solve an easy real-life problem, such as deciding what to have for dinner or where to go for an evening outing.

Step 2: Using Family Problem Solving at Home

The final step is solving a real-life family problem. Have the ***Family Problem Solving*** chart available to family members while trying to resolve more difficult issues. It's important that family members go through each step very carefully, one at a time.

 TROUBLESHOOTING TIP
Make sure that your child understands that all problems are not open to this give-and-take approach. The parent is still in charge, and with some issues the parent holds veto power. Do not use family problem solving unless you really are open to compromise or negotiation.

Strategy 3: Managing Family Conflict

Step 1: Helping Family Members Recognize Family Conflict

Ask family members to participate in a family meeting at a time everyone agrees to and when everyone is in a good mood, to work on getting along better. The first task for the family is to recognize the signals that tell them they are having conflict. All family members should help create examples of signals while another person writes them down. Here are a few examples of family conflict signals:

Personal Body Signals within Family Members

- Breathing rate increases
- Flushed face color
- Heart rate increases
- Muscle tension increases
- Sweating increases

Personal Thought Signals within Family Members

- "She's making me mad."
- "He is so unfair."
- "I hate her!"
- "I wish he would move out of the house."
- "I wish she were dead."
- "I'm going to hit him."

Family Behavior Signals between Family Members

- Raised voices
- Put-down verbalizations
- Angry facial expressions
- Interrupting
- Angry body postures

PRACTICE EXERCISE

It is helpful to practice recognizing family conflict signals. Begin with neutral and easy problems before trying more difficult problems. Have the family act out disagreements, such as what to have for dinner or what to watch on TV. Pretend there is a blow-up. Then ask family members to recount the family conflict signals from the role play.

After family members become adept at recognizing conflict, proceed to learning how to manage it.

Step 2: Learning and Practicing Family Conflict Management Skills

During a family meeting, discuss the **family cool-down** procedure, which can be used whenever family conflict arises. The family cool-down procedure involves family members separating from each other for a few minutes to calm down by themselves:

- Family members should agree ahead of time that any one of them can call for a family cool-down.

- Once a family cool-down is called, everyone separates for an agreed-upon amount of time, such as 5 or 10 minutes.

- Then each family member practices dealing with his or her own anger and frustration.

Here are a few ways to practice calming down during the separation phase:

- Breathe deeply.

- Tense and relax your muscles.

- Make helpful statements to yourself, such as: "I'm not going to let her get to me," "I'm going to try to stay cool," "I'll try to say it in a different way to get my point across to him."

- Do something to briefly distract yourself, such as step outside, look at the newspaper, or watch TV for a few minutes.

After family members have calmed down, come back together and use effective family communication and problem-solving skills to resolve whatever triggered the conflict.

The **Family Cool-Down** chart (at the end of this chapter) provides an easy plan to follow. It might help for family members to have this chart handy when they try to reduce family conflict.

 PRACTICE EXERCISE
Go back to the same scenarios practiced in Step 1. Ask the family again to pretend to have disagreements, such as what to have for dinner or what to watch on TV. Pretend there is a blowup, someone calls for a family cool-down, everyone separates for a few minutes to cool off, and then everyone reassembles to work it out.

Step 3: Using Family Conflict Management Skills at Home

After all members of the family have learned the skills in practice, they can use them when real-life family conflict happens. **It may be difficult, but when family conflict erupts, try to guide your family through each step, one by one.** After the

> ## PUTTING IT ALL TOGETHER
>
> Once you all have it down, it is okay to use family communication skills while trying to solve family problems with everyone staying calm. Try to use good communication while discussing and working through problems as they come up.

family has cooled off, try to discuss and resolve the original problem that caused the conflict. It may be helpful to post the *Family Cool-Down* chart for family members to refer to when a conflict or argument arises.

Achieving Success with Family Interactions

Family interaction skills involve communicating, solving problems, and resolving conflicts during daily family activities. This chapter provides strategies for helping your family learn to use those important skills. To follow through, periodically review the *Parent Checklist for Family Interactions* at the end of this chapter or set your own goals to attain with the *Parenting Goals* form at the end of Chapter 3.

It takes time to break old family habits, and there is a risk of relapse. You need to be **persistent** and **consistent** (i.e., PERCON) in applying these skills-building strategies every day until they work. Sometimes this takes weeks or months.

Parent Checklist for Family Interactions

Name: _____ **Date:** _____

In the blanks below, indicate a score for **how well** you make use of that parenting behavior at this time.

Not too well	Okay	Very well
1	2	3

Parent's Efforts in Promoting Family Communication Skills

A. _____ Reviewing and practicing family communication skills

B. _____ Guiding the family to use the family communication skills at home, including reviewing the charts

Parent's Efforts in Promoting Family Problem-Solving Skills

C. _____ Reviewing and practicing family problem-solving skills

D. _____ Guiding the family to use the family problem-solving skills at home, including reviewing the charts

Parent's Efforts in Promoting Family Conflict Management Skills

E. _____ Reviewing and practicing family conflict resolution skills

F. _____ Guiding the family to use the family conflict resolution skills at home, including reviewing the charts

Family Communication Skills

DON'Ts

- Long lectures or "sermons"

- Blaming (e.g., "You need to stop _____," "It's your fault")

- Vague statements (e.g., "Shape up," "Knock it off," "I don't like that")

- Asking negative questions (e.g., "Why do you do that?" or "How many times must I tell you?")

- Poor listening—looking away, silent treatment, crossing arms, etc.

- Interrupting others

- Not showing that you understand someone

- Put-downs (e.g., "You're worthless," "I'm sick of you"), threats, and so forth

- Yelling, screaming, and so forth

- Sarcasm

- Going from topic to topic

- Bringing up old issues, past behavior

- Keeping feelings inside

- Scowling facial expression

- "Mind reading" or assuming you know what other people think

DOs

- Brief statements of 10 words or less

- "I" statements (e.g., "I feel _____ when _____")

- Direct and specific statements (e.g., "Stop teasing your sister [brother]," "I really don't like when you _____")

- Be specific about what you want (e.g., "Do the dishes now," "Please talk calmly")

- Active listening—good eye contact, leaning forward, nodding, etc.

- Let person completely state his or her thoughts before stating yours

- Paraphrase what the other person said to you

- Constructive comments (e.g., "I'm concerned about your grades," "Something is bothering me; can we discuss it?")

- Neutral/natural tone of voice

- Say what you mean, be specific and straightforward

- Stay on one topic

- Focusing on here and now

- Verbally expressing feelings

- Neutral facial expressions

- Let people speak for themselves; ask questions to make sure you understand

My Family Communication Goals

Name: _____ **Date and time:** _____

Indicate which family communication "DOs" you will be working on below. Designate a time period for using this chart. At the end of the designated time period, rate how well you accomplished your goals. It may be helpful to get feedback from other family members as to how well they think you are accomplishing your goals.

Self-Awareness Monitoring

1. I am working on increasing family communication DOs of:

2. How well did I accomplish my goal(s)? (Circle one.)

1	2	3	4	5
Not at all	A little	Okay	Pretty well	Great

Family Members' Feedback (optional)

3. How well did family members think I accomplished my goal(s)? (Circle one.)

1	2	3	4	5
Not at all	A little	Okay	Pretty well	Great

Comments: _____

_____

_____

_____

_____

Family Problem Solving

1. **Stop!! What is the problem we are having?**

   - Try to avoid blaming individuals.

   - Focus on how family members are interacting and causing problems together.

   - State specifically what the problem is so that everyone agrees.

2. **What are some plans we can use?**

   - Think of as many alternative plans as possible.

   - Don't evaluate or criticize any family member's ideas.

   - Don't discuss any one solution until you have generated many alternatives.

3. **What is the best plan we could use?**

   - Think of what would happen if the family used each of the alternatives.

   - Think about how each alternative would make each family member feel.

   - Decide which alternative is most likely to succeed and make most family members feel okay.

   - Reach an agreement by as many family members as possible.

4. **Put the plan into effect.**

   - Try the plan as well as the family can.

   - Don't criticize or say, "I told you so."

5. **Did our plan work?**

   - Evaluate the plan.

   - Determine whether everyone is satisfied with the way the problem was solved.

   - If the solution didn't work, repeat the entire family problem-solving process.

Try to stay focused on the here and now. Do not bring up old issues when trying to do family problem solving.

Family Cool-Down

1. Are we too angry at each other?

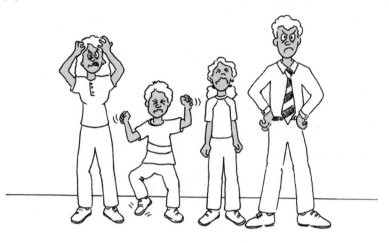

2. Briefly separate to cool down.

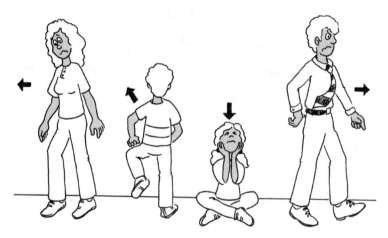

3. Come back together to solve the problem.

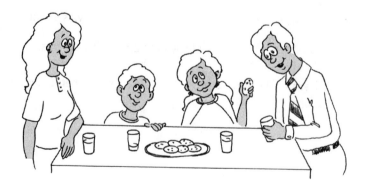

From *Skills Training for Struggling Kids.* Copyright 2013 by The Guilford Press.

Family Cool-Down

1. **Are we too angry at each other?**

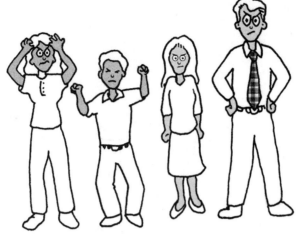

2. **Briefly separate to cool down.**

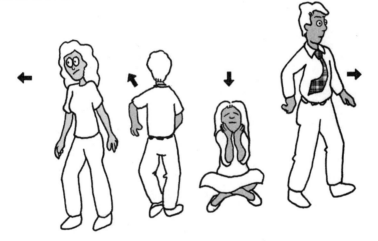

3. **Come back together to solve the problem.**

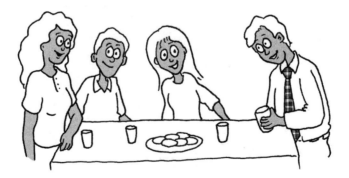

Resources

Many of these organizations offer valuable information for parents on health, education, and mental health issues. They often also provide ways to locate appropriate therapists, to get your child's educational needs met, and to find local parenting and family groups. I have included resources for websites in the United States and Canada, the United Kingdom, and Australia/New Zealand.

American Academy of Pediatrics
www.aap.org

American Academy of Child and Adolescent Psychiatry (AACAP)
www.aacap.org

American Association for Marriage and Family Therapy (AAMFT)
www.aamft.org

American Psychological Association (APA)
www.apa.org

Association for Behavioral and Cognitive Therapies (ABCT)
www.abct.org

Canadian Pediatric Society
www.cps.ca/english

Children and Adults with Attention-Deficit/Hyperactivity Disorder (CHADD)
www.chadd.org

Council for Exceptional Children
www.cec.sped.org

Early Childhood Australia
www.earlychildhoodaustralia.org. au

Family Education
www.familyeducation.com

Intervention Central
www.interventioncentral.org

LD OnLine
www.ldonline.org

Learning Disabilities Association of America
www.ldanatl.org

Learning Disabilities Association of Canada
www.ldac-acta.ca

National Alliance on Mental Illness (NAMI)
www.nami.org

National Association of School Psychologists (NASP)
www.nasponline.org

National Center for Learning Disabilities
www.ncld.org

National Institute of Child Health and Human Development (NICHD)
www.nichd.nih.gov

Smart Kids with Learning Disabilities
www.smartkidswithld.org

Specific Learning Disabilities Federation (SPELD) New Zealand
www.speld.org.nz

Thanet ADDers
www.adders.org/thanet.htm

Index

About the Author

Michael L. Bloomquist, PhD, a child psychologist, is Associate Professor of Psychiatry at the University of Minnesota, where he conducts research and trains practitioners. He is the author of a related book for mental health professionals, *The Practitioner Guide to Skills Training for Struggling Kids.* Dr. Bloomquist has worked with struggling kids and teens and their families for over 25 years. He and his wife are the proud parents of two sons.